The Truth About **HORMONES**

D1386261

The Truth About

HORMONES

Vivienne Parry

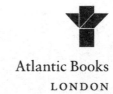

Atlantic Books
LONDON

Published in Trade Paperback in Great Britain in 2005 by Atlantic Books
Atlantic Books is an imprint of Grove Atlantic Ltd.

10 9 8 7 6 5 4 3 2 1

A CIP catalogue record for this book is available from the British Library.
ISBN 1 84354 428 8

Set in 11.5/14.25pt Monotype Sabon
Designed by Nicky Barneby @ Barneby Ltd
Printed in Great Britain by William Clowes Ltd, Beccles, Suffolk

Atlantic Books
An imprint of Grove Atlantic Ltd
Ormond House
26–27 Boswell Street
London
WC1N 3JZ

CONTENTS

ACKNOWLEDGEMENTS

Very special thanks to the following: Professor Eric Thomas, who gave up female hormones to be a fabulous Vice Chancellor and Professor Clive Coen, a fabulous neuroendrocrinologist, who each read my manuscript and offered much helpful comment; Professor Steve Franks, reproductive endocrinologist, for lending me several huge volumes from his hormone library, as well as for his thoughtful advice and support; Professor David Purdie, master of HRT and the spoken word for his comments on the menopause chapter, Dr Jo Marsden for her help with breast cancer; and physiologist Professor Michael Rennie, who made sense of insulin and growth hormone for me and who, when I apologized for making him read his subject transcribed for toddlers, came back with the words I want engraved on my tombstone: 'Your demotic is sufficiently racy not to be insulting.' Only a scientist eh?

A special thank you to Tom Parkhill and the Society for Endocrinology who were unfailingly helpful in offering their contacts and knowledge and who made it possible for me to attend the International Congress of Endrocrinology 2004 in Lisbon. They also read the manuscript with good grace, despite being surrounded by hormones.

Many doctors and scientists were incredibly generous with their time: the sperm men, Professor Chris Barratt and Dr Allan Pacey, lactation specialist Professor Peter Howie, the ever patient Dr Alan Johnson of the Centre for Ecology and Hydrology, Wallingford, Professor Roger Gosden, Professor Shlomo Melmed, the sveltest obesity expert I know, Professor Steve Bloom, Professor Howard

Jacobs, Blakemores, père et fille (Professor Colin and Dr Sarah), Professor Sir Iain Chalmers, Dr Margaret Rees, Sir Dr Chris Flowers, Dr John Gilbody of Wyeth, Dr John Ashby of Syngenta, Dr Mark Lythgoe, Prof Neil Gittoes and Professor John Russell, come to mind in particular but there were many more that I bored to death with a constant stream of questions. To all of you, thank you. And what would I have done without the support, contacts and gossip from staff at the Science Media Centre, MRC, Nature News Service and the Environment Agency? I was also indulged by many of the science correspondents, including Tim Radford, Nigel Hawkes and Mark Henderson as I expounded my wilder hormone theories over a glass or three; and cosseted by John Adams, a professor of geography, who runs a course on statistics for the mathematically challenged. His attempt to instil understanding of standard deviation was largely successful.

When I last wrote a book, a decade ago, I swore I wouldn't do another one. The combination of Toby Mundy of Atlantic Books – as inspirational, enthusiastic and talented a publisher as you could hope to find – and my agent Pat Kavanagh, changed my mind. Dr Louisa Joyner edited this book and was a joy to work with, as were all the staff at Atlantic, including Jane Robertson, the copy editor whose family probably all got socks as presents because I drove Jane witless in the week before Christmas. I feel very lucky to have found them.

I owe a great deal to my family who endured me locking myself away for too long and for my patient and loving friends whom I neglected horribly while I wrote this, and for whom the excuse 'It's my hormones' wore a little thin. Finally, this book is for my father. Had they known more about hormones thirty years ago, he might have been alive today, hopefully to be proud.

Vivienne Parry
Muswell Hill 2005

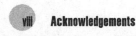

INTRODUCTION

Hormones rule your world. They control your growth, your weight, your metabolism, your fertility and water balance. They initiate and regulate life changes like puberty and menopause, they have a hand in the speed of ageing, whether you want sex or not (and even whether you enjoy it), and who you fall in love with. Their effects may occur in seconds and be over in a flash, or take months and last for thirty years. They control your mood and your emotions too, especially those that grip you in the most visceral way – fear, anger, love.

Whatever your age or gender, whether you are petulant, cranky, spotty, forgetful, angry or just a little out of sorts, the odds are that someone is going to tell you 'It's your hormones'. Irritatingly, there's a good chance they're right.

The word 'hormone' appears in the media almost every day. Challenged, people will hazard that testosterone is one, that the pill contains them and maybe that fish are changing sex because of them. This book will explain how hormones work and introduce the myriad ways that they control your life and the controversy and outrage that so often attend them.

This book isn't a manual for those with hormone-based conditions like diabetes, thyroid disease or infertility, for whom there are already many practical guides. It is an introduction to a secret empire of stunning complexity and elegance, and will attempt to set out the truth about hormones.

Hormones are the slaves of one of the body's two internal communication systems. The nervous system carries messages from the brain that are transmitted throughout the body by electrical stimuli. The hormone system – more properly known as the endocrine system – is much slower, and uses the blood as its medium for communication and chemicals – hormones – as its messengers. To compare the two systems is to compare a high-speed rail network with canals, or snail mail to e-mail.

Hormones are molecules with a very long history. Even the simplest of animals needed to communicate what was going on outside its body to each of its cells inside. Without some form of internal communication, how could it coordinate a response that would ensure its survival? Come to that, how could the animal function as one organism, without some means of enabling all its constituent parts to talk to each other?

Chemical messengers work by travelling to a cell with an instruction to do something. Once they reach their target, the molecules of hormone find unique docking bays, called receptors, and deliver their message. At first it was thought that hormones in 'higher' animals were produced solely by special ductless glands, called endocrine glands, like the thyroid or the ovaries, and that each of these glands, with its specialized hormones, worked in isolation to do a specific job. It was then realized that the glands, which also include the testicles, the pancreas and the adrenal glands on top of each kidney, worked together, with one of them, the pituitary (positioned at the base of the brain and just behind your eyes), acting as the conductor that orchestrated them all. It is now known that the master gland is actually the brain itself, specifically a part of it called the hypothalamus, from which the pituitary dangles by a little stalk, and that lots of organs act as endocrine glands – including the placenta and gut – and that many if not all tissues including fat and muscle, produce hormones. Hormones, which were once believed to number no more than a couple of dozen, are today counted in the hundreds.

When people talk about their hormones, they talk about them in the abstract, as if they were something over which they had no control. It's true we have no say in the genes we acquire, which contain the instructions for the various elements of the endocrine system. It's true that hormones are a bit like breathing in that they work independently of conscious thought. But in another sense we do control them: it is our actions that drive them; they are the body's response to our conscious activities, whether it is running a marathon, falling in love or eating Christmas lunch.

Given the complexity of the endocrine system, it is perhaps not suprising that it can go wrong. Indeed, from the earliest times the conditions caused by having too little or too much of a particular hormone were remarkable enough and common enough to attract the interest of enquiring minds. These conditions included gigantism, caused by an excess of growth hormone; the growth of a big lump on the neck called a goitre, symptomatic of too little thyroid hormone; and the wasting, decline and rapid death of those with diabetes. The removal of one set of endocrine glands – the testicles – were understood to be linked to changes in body shape and function in both humans and animals. Despite this understanding the history of hormones is a recent one, with the actual word hormone being coined only a century ago, in June 1905.

The pivotal figure in the history of hormones was Charles Eduoard Brown-Séquard. British by birth, but French by upbringing, he was a world-famous neurologist of the Victorian era. In 1855, he established that the adrenal glands, which sit one atop each kidney and produce, among other hormones, the stress hormone cortisol, were essential to life. He also refined the concept of 'internal secretion' – the idea that organs inside the body could produce substances which travel around the body in the bloodstream and affect the function of other organs.

However, it was to be another forty years before the word hormone was coined. In 1902 William Bayliss and Ernest Starling, physiologists working at University College London, were the first to discover and name one of these mysterious 'internal secretions', a hormone produced in the gut called secretin. Sir William Hardy suggested using the term hormone, which means 'to arouse or excite', or, as some Greek scholars would have it, 'to urge'. The first recorded use of the word was in the annual Croonian lecture to the Royal College of Physicians, given by Starling, in June 1905. Rival groups of doctors had proposed a different name – 'harmazones' from the Greek 'to regulate' – but, perhaps luckily, given that a 'harmazone' sounds like something you should suck for a sore throat, 'hormone' was preferred.

Hormones, however, were already notorious. In 1889, Brown-Séquard, now seventy-two years old, was back in France where he had taken up the distinguished position of Professor of Medicine at the Collège de France. On 1 June, he stood before the Society of Biology in Paris and announced his own rejuvenations. The elixir? The gound-up testicles, semen and blood of guinea pigs and a dog, extracted with water, filtered, diluted and injected daily. After just eight injections, Brown-Séquard said he felt less fatigued, could lift heavier weights than before and no longer needed laxatives. The effect of this announcement from such an eminent doctor was electrifying.

While Brown-Séquard's rejuvenating fluid was greeted with scepticism in Britain, in America it had a sensational impact. The world and his wife, or rather the world and his mistress he would like to service, beat a path to his door, clamouring for his organ extracts. Within weeks, testicular extracts were being given to patients to cure everything from high blood pressure to headaches. By the following year, over 1,200 doctors were giving this 'elixir' to their patients and it sparked a craze for 'oganotherapy' – the concept of giving extracts of a particular organ to cure problems associated with the same organ. It was soon to encompass not just testicular extracts but almost every body organ – even 'grey matter' – suitable for treatment of nervous diseases.

The testicular extracts had no effect, because testosterone (the 'rejuvenating' hormone Brown-Séquard had been seeking) was not soluble in water. They were also extremely dangerous and it was likely there were many deaths caused by infection or extreme allergic reation. While their appeal gradually receded, organotherapy endured for another fifty years in various forms, including the widespread use of implanted animal testicles during the 1930s by the so-called 'gland grafters', such as John Brinkley in the US and Serge Voronoff in Europe.

So, from the outset, hormones were mired in quackery and controversy and since then have never been far from the front pages of newspapers. It took a Nobel prize in 1923, awarded following Frederick Banting and Charles Best's discovery of insulin, to finally mark endocrinology – the study of hormones – as a science worthy of respectable academic study. Despite giant leaps forward in the science (endocrinology has garnered a quarter of all Nobel prizes for Physiology or Medicine since 1970), there are still the two same diverging paths taken today as there were in 1905: that taken by academic medicine and that travelled by the quacks and charlatans peddling eternal youth, better sex and beautiful bodies.

CHAPTER ONE

A BLUFFER'S GUIDE TO HORMONES

Hormones have an elegance and matchless wonder about them that is little known or understood. Part of the reason for this is that the language of hormones is so confusing with numerous acronyms and a tendency to call the same thing by many different names. The stress hormone cortisol, for example, is also referred to as hydro-cortisone, there are variants such as cortisone and corticosterone – which are essentially one and the same thing to all but very particular chemists. Not only that, but cortisol can quite correctly be called a steroid, as well as a glucocorticoid, or even a corticosteroid, depending on the context. Such confusion can make hormone-ology appear impenetrable at first, but, let me reassure you, it's basically easy. This is not string theory or mobile phone contracts.

To start with the basics, 'endocrine' means secretion within, and endocrine glands do just that. They produce secretions within the gland and rely on the blood to take what they have produced to the rest of the body. Compare and contrast with the so-called exocrine glands, like digestive glands or sweat glands, which all have ducts to pipe their secretions out to the specific spot where they're needed, like the gut or your armpit. Another (older) name for the endocrine glands is the ductless glands.

The study of hormones is called endocrinology, and someone who works with hormones is called an endocrinologist. The whole system of glands and hormones in the body is called the endocrine system. The endocrine system coordinates activity inside the body, regulates development throughout life and helps the body adapt to change outside the body. It controls things like reproduction, metabolism and growth. It can also have a profound effect on mood and emotion – which we are all too aware of. The endocrine system is one of two major communication systems in the body, the other being the nervous system. They are closely linked and indeed *neuro*-endocrinology, the study of hormone and nerve interactions, is one of the largest and fastest expanding areas of endocrinology.

As an illustration of the radically different speeds of the two systems, consider colour change. Watch a chameleon, octopus or squid change colour. It's utterly dazzling, a lightning-fast moving colour display, reflecting not just the animal's background coloration, but seemingly its mood too. If an octopus is angered this is instantly reflected in its hue. That's the nervous system at work, for it mediates colour change in these animals. Consider a frog – its colour change system is hormone-driven. The outer layers of its skin has cells, called melanophores, containing dots of melanin pigment. If the pigment dots are clumped together, at the centre of melanophore, the animal will appear to be a light colour but if the pigment dots are dispersed throughout, the animal will seem to be a much lighter coloured creature. The dispersal of these pigment dots is under the influence of a pituitary hormone, melanocyt-stimulating hormone (MSH). Compared to the nervous system, however, it is very slow. If you put a light-coloured frog in a dark box, it will be several hours before it is well on the way to becoming a dark one. The entire light to dark process may take up to a day.

So hormones can be produced in those ductless glands, released into the blood, and have an effect on a specific tissue, far away from the gland. The upshot may be to gear things up (stimulatory) or damp them down (inhibitory). When they arrive at a cell, some change takes place in the cell, according to the message received.

Working from head to toe, the classic endocrine glands are the anterior pituitary (in the base of the brain), the thyroid and parathyroids (in the neck), the pancreas, two adrenal glands (which sit on the top of the kidneys) and two testes or ovaries. All of these glands manufacture particular hormones, some of which will be very familiar, like insulin from the pancreas and testosterone from the testes. A common feature of all these classical endocrine glands is an excellent blood supply, for blood is their main channel of communication.

The grand vizier of the hormone empire is the hypothalamus, a region of the brain which is roughly behind your eyes, and hormones are the slaves of the system, chemical messengers too small to be seen, which carry instructions to cells all over the body.

At any one time there are thousands, perhaps millions, of messages in the blood being carried by hormones. The endocrine system is one of constant change: it always strikes me as a bit like the most perfect civil service, responsive to every little nuance from every last citizen, constantly receiving messages about the state of the nation, and constantly reacting with new instructions so as to attain perfect governance and order. However, unlike real governments, where civil servants in Trade and Industry never talk to those in Health, every single department is involved and cross-linked, with each knowing what every other department is doing – and adding its own addendum to the instruction if necessary.

That grand vizier – the hypothalamus – sits at the base of the brain and is in charge of hormone production, although its ultimate master is the rest of the brain. For such an important gland, the hypothalamus is incredibly small – less than a lump of sugar.

The pea-sized pituitary (the most important of those classic glands) dangles from the hypothalamus by a little stalk. Inside the stalk is a complex network of blood vessels called the hypophyseal portal system. The hypothalamus produces two types of regulating hormone, releasing ones and inhibiting ones, all of which act on the pituitary. The portal system within the stalk carries these command hormones from the hypothalamus to the front end of the pituitary, which is called the anterior pituitary. The back end – the posterior pituitary or neurohypophysis – is more of a storage area, particularly for vasopressin, which controls water balance, and oxytocin, the hormone of love and birth, both of which are manufactured in the hypothalamus. The pituitary and hypothalamus effectively function together as one unit, known as the hypothalamic-pituitary axis.

The function of the hypothalamus is as a translation *and* command unit, receiving input from the brain and then sending out appropriate messages, sometimes by nerve impulses, and sometimes by employing hormones via the pituitary gland. The hypothalamus is in control because it is wired directly into its ultimate master – the brain. Everything you experience or perceive – from a bear running down the corridor at work, to a hot romance, to seeing an empty shelf where you expected food to be – the brain, via the senses, gets to know first and it has to make decisions about what to do next. The brain can parcel out response messages via the body's two communication networks, the nervous system and the endocrine system. For an almost instant response, the nervous system is used; where a slower response will do, it's the endocrine alternative. But there is also a third way – using nerves to stimulate the production of hormones. Three endocrine glands secrete their hormones only in response to nerve stimuli: the adrenal medulla, which pours out adrenaline and noradrenaline, the hormones that prepare you for 'fight or flight'; the pineal gland, which secretes melatonin, hormone of sleep; and the posterior pituitary, which is the warehouse for vasopressin and oxytocin. This response is not quite as instant as that produced by the nerves alone, but nevertheless a chain reaction can occur in seconds.

How Does It All Work?

First, let me say something about terminology. The word 'trophic' ('tropic' in the US) at the end of a hormone word makes that word an adjective. The root word before it describes the target of that hormone – so 'gonadotrophic' means acting on the gonads;

The Truth About Hormones

'neurotrophic', acting on the nerves; 'somatotrophic', acting on the body and so on. The word 'trophin' ('tropin' in the US) at the end of the word makes it a noun. This means that the hormone has a releasing effect on another system – although 'unleashing' is a more appropriate word than 'releasing'.

Now, let's consider the release of thyroid hormones as an illustration of how hormones work. Hormones tend to come in pairs or groups of three. There's the hormone itself and then there's a mate (or two) involved in its release or inhibition. Quite often the hormone regulates itself, in that when a certain level of the hormone in the bloodstream is reached, this in itself prevents more being secreted.

The hypothalamus is bathed in circulating blood, and when blood levels of thyroid hormone are low, the hypothalamus produces thyrotrophin releasing hormone, usually known as TRH. TRH travels down the stalk connecting the hypothalamus to the pituitary, to the front section, anterior pituitary, and delivers its message: 'More thyroid hormone needed'. The pituitary obliges, releasing thyroid stimulating hormone (TSH), which travels through the bloodstream to the thyroid gland itself, in the neck. There, in response to the message delivered by TSH, more thyroid hormone is produced.

It's the next stage that is the key to understanding how hormones operate. The thyroid will go on producing thyroid hormones until it is told to stop. If thyroid hormones are over-produced and their levels in the bloodstream become too high, the 'levels too high' message is received by the hypothalamus and the amount of TRH being produced is then decreased. As a result, the anterior pituitary gets the message, 'Slow down on thyroid production'. This is called negative feedback. If on the other hand, levels of thyroid hormone fall too low, the hypothalamus produces more thyrotrophin releasing hormone, begetting more thyroid stimulating hormone, and more thyroid hormone once again. Negative feedback systems are a very common feature of hormone function.

So we have the hypothalamus – which is part of the brain – producing releasing and inhibiting hormones in response to signals from outside the body and from signals within the body. Here are the ones you are most likely to come across.

Thyrotrophin releasing hormone (TRH) controls thyroid stimulating hormone and thence the production of thyroid hormones.

Growth hormone releasing hormone (GHRH) and its partner *somatostatin* which inhibit both growth hormone and thyroid stimulating hormone.

Gonadotrophin releasing hormone (GnRH) stimulates follicle stimulating hormone and luteinising hormone secretion (the hormones that control testis or ovary).

Corticotrophin releasing hormone or factor (CRH) stimulates adrenocorticotrophic hormone (ACTH), which in turn controls production of stress hormones.

These hormones act on the anterior pituitary, the front part of the pituitary gland which dangles by a stalk from underneath the hypothalamus. Four of the anterior pituitary's hormones control specific endocrine glands. *Luteinising hormone* (LH) and *follicle stimulating hormone* (FSH) act on the gonads – that is, the ovaries or testicles. These hormones are the same in men and women, even though the target organs are clearly different. *Thyroid stimulating hormone* controls the thyroid gland and *adrenocorticotrophin* (ACTH) the adrenal glands. The anterior pituitary also produces two hormones directly: *growth hormone*, which has effects throughout the body, but mainly on bone and soft tissue, and *prolactin*, the hormone of lactation which acts on the breasts to produce milk.

Let's look at the principal hormones produced by each of the endocrine glands.

The **ovaries** are the main site for the production of oestrogens, of which there are several different types. *Oestrone* and *oestradiol* are the best known. Oestrogens vary in potency – oestrone, for instance, is relatively weak, whereas oestradiol is the more potent. The ovaries also produce the hormone progesterone, which comes in a single variety and which, like the oestrogens, is a steroid hormone.

The **testicles** secrete *testosterone*. You may be surprised to know that the work of producing male hormones is shared by another pair of endocrine glands, the adrenals, although these produce far smaller quantities of male hormones. Testosterone is, like oestrogen, a steroid hormone.

The **adrenals** are called the fight or flight glands and are all about keeping the body going in times of stress. They are a pair of small triangular glands, one atop each kidney. The cortex, or outer portion, of the adrenal is divided into three layers, all producing steroid hormones, which, because they come from the cortex are collectively called corticosteroids. The outer layer produces *aldosterone*, which plays a vital role in the control of blood pressure and in the regulation of the salts potassium and sodium in the blood and tissues. Aldosterone is a mineralocorticoid (a word that describes its job of salt balance) but it is also called a corticosteroid – because it comes from the cortex. The middle layer produces *cortisol*, a glucocorticoid (another job word, which describes its role in regulating energy levels) and the hormone most familiar to us as the classic stress hormone. The inner, thinnest layer produces androgens – male hormones – in both men and women. Finally the inner core of the gland, the medulla, produces *adrenaline* and *noradrenaline*, which are all members of a family of chemicals called catecholamines including *dopamine*. These are not steroid hormones like the rest of the hormones produced by the adrenal glands, but are more similar to the hormones of the thyroid gland. Noradrenaline and dopamine have a critical role as very specific sorts of chemical messengers, which do not carry messages through the bloodstream but between one nerve cell and another.

When acting as transmitters the catecholamine carry messages across the gap between one nerve ending and the next. Neurotransmitters are released from nerve endings in response to electrical impulses travelling down the nerve. Nerve system messaging is a bit like an electrically driven relay race, with the baton being exchanged in the gap between one nerve and the next. Adrenaline and noradrenaline are both a neurotransmitter and a hormone.

(Confusingly, Americans call adrenaline and noradrenaline, epinephrine and norepinephrine respectively. European terminology is used throughout this book but you can find the American forms in some of the references cited at the end of the book . You may also see the word 'adrenalin' and wonder whether it is the same as 'adrenaline'. It is. The correct spelling is with an 'e' as in cate-cholamine.)

The **thyroid** is the largest endocrine organ. It sits in the neck, just below the voice box and has two lobes, one on either side of your windpipe, joined by a strap of tissue which gives it the shape of a butterfly. It produces two thyroid hormones: very large quantities of *thyroxine* (T4) and much smaller amounts of *triiodothyronine* (T3). When thyroxine reaches its target tissues it is converted to the biologically much more potent T3, so you could call T4 a pro-hormone. Unlike other hormones, thyroid hormone levels are kept remarkably constant – rather like the way the body keeps glucose levels constant. To make its hormones, the thyroid needs iodine, which it gets from food. If there is no iodine available to manufacture T4 and T3, the body will need to draw on its stores, thus keeping levels steady, no matter what the fluctuation in food supplies.

The thyroid controls metabolism and energy balance. If the body doesn't have enough thyroid, it slows right down. If it has too much, you feel like you're on fast-forward all the time. Although thyroxine is a hormone of metabolism in humans, it is the hormone of metamorphosis in amphibians. You can demonstrate this very easily if you happen to have a bowlful of tadpoles handy. Just put a thyroxine tablet, intended for someone who has a poorly functioning thyroid, into the water. The tadpoles will miraculously change into tiny frogs almost overnight.

There are four **parathyroids**, two behind either side of the thyroid in the neck. They are small – pea sized – but significant in that they regulate calcium levels. Without calcium there would be no muscle contraction or nerve transmissions and no blood clotting. The parathyroids aren't under the direct control of the hypothalamus, but can be thought of as being an elite gland squad. They can direct how much calcium is removed from the body's stores in the bones and how much is reabsorbed via the kidneys and intestine if blood levels of calcium fall too low. The hormone is *parathyroid hormone*. One further hormone closely involved in calcium balance within the body is *calcitonin*, another hormone of the thyroid gland.

The **pancreas** has two main jobs. It is a leaf-shaped organ that lies behind the stomach. About 98 per cent of it is made of tissue which secretes digestive enzymes. It is said to be an exocrine gland, because it pipes its secretions away through a duct – the pancreatic duct – into the duodenum. However, within this exocrine tissue are nests of tens of thousands of little of hormone-producing cells – the so-called islets of Langerhans. Thus 98 per cent of the pancreas is an exocrine digestive gland, but 2 per cent of it is an endocrine gland involved in regulation of the body's fuel system.

One cell type within these islets secretes the hormone *glucagon* and the other sort secretes *insulin*. When sugar levels are high, insulin is released; when it is low, glucagon is released. These two hormones reach every part of the body and affect almost every tissue, for the body's efficient running depends on glucose being kept within a very tight range – never too much, never too little. As constant as possible is what the body likes best.

If the islets are destroyed – as they are by the immune systems of those people who develop insulin-dependent diabetes – blood glucose levels rise astronomically. Even though the person's blood contains huge amounts of glucose, without insulin's help the body is unable to use it as fuel.

How is insulin controlled? Does the hypothalamus have a role in this particular scenario? There is no direct insulin regulator produced by the hypothalamus or pituitary. However, noradrenaline, cortisol, growth hormone and the thyroid hormones all play an important part in controlling blood sugar – and all of these are under the dominion of the hypothalamus.

When Is A Gland Not A Gland?

Originally the definition of a classic endocrine gland was that it secreted a hormone into the blood, which had an effect on a distant tissue. It was convenient to think of endocrine glands as being specific organs, but as more become known about hormones, it was realized that this was an over-simplification. For instance, the pancreas is a gland within a gland, because only patches of tissue within the pancreas – the islets of Langerhans – produce hormones. Although some hormone-secreting cells are collected together in glands, there are others which are just single cells found within some other organ, like the gut, liver or the skin. The hormones released from these single cells may act on themselves (so-called autocrine hormones) or they may affect nearby cells (paracrine hormones). One example is *secretin*, produced in the gut, another hormone which has a role in sugar regulation.

The original definition of a hormone as something which had, as its target a 'distant organ' proved problematic, for it became clear that hormones didn't have to travel – they could act locally. The whole concept of what constituted a gland also became stretched. The great discovery of the last thirty years has been that far from there being just a few obvious endocrine glands, and twenty or so major hormones, many tissues act as endocrine glands in their own right, producing hormones unique to that tissue. Fat cells, for instance, are now known to produce the hormone *leptin*. Muscles produce *IGF-2*. The placenta is a hormone-producing organ. With the acceptance of this concept has come the realization that there are literally hundreds of hormones.

Many hormones are secreted either in a cyclical fashion (for instance, once a month as with female reproductive hormones) or in a pulsed way (like gonadotrophin releasing hormone, which is released in bursts, every ninety minutes or so). Hormone production varies during a twenty-four-hour period too. For example, testosterone levels are highest first thing in the morning. Growth hormone and the milk-producing hormone prolactin are released during sleep. This has implications for attempts to measure hormones. Single measurements are rarely that instructive, for they are simply snapshots at a particular moment in time. Usually urine collection over twenty-four hours will be needed to give an accurate assessment of hormone levels.

If you look at the back of medical textbooks, you will see what are called 'reference tables', which give the top and bottom ranges of values considered usual for levels of various body chemicals. There are also reference ranges for hormones, but what distinguishes many of them is how wide they are. There is an optimum level for good health but the important thing is that it's what is optimum for you that counts, not what is good for someone else. We are all uniquely hormoned. Nowadays a number of organizations offer to test the levels of your hormones for 'optimum functioning'. The usual practice is to pronounce you 'deficient' in some of them, before selling you what they say is required for you to reach the 'right' level, as defined by them. This is marketing, not science. We are not yet clever enough to know what is the best individual level of hormones for people in good health, and those that tell you they do know are to be avoided.

Receptors

All hormones have a final destination – an individual cell which the hormone has to instruct – and so another key part of the endocrine system is receptors. The surfaces of cells are covered with these receptors, which you can think of as docking bays. They are needed because most hormones can't pass through the cell membrane, despite the fact that their message needs to be delivered to the nucleus inside the cell. They lock into 'their' receptor on the outside of the cell and then a strange thing happens. It's like a celebrity walking into your local, setting off a chain of gossip inside the pub, in which one person tells another, who tells two more and so on until there's nobody who doesn't know that Madonna has just bought a half of lager. However, dissemination of information needs to be translated into action. It's as if it were understood that when Madonna appears, a specific set-piece action has to take place: the landlord is informed, he phones the *News of the World*, who sends round a photographer so that his boozer will be on the front page. The equivalent in the cell is that of the so-called second messenger system, in which other molecules carry the news that a hormone has docked to many other molecules inside the cell, as well as telling the nucleus what needs to be done. This ripple effect means that only tiny amounts of hormone are required for a major response.

Receptors are also highly selective. They provide a specific docking bay for every hormone. Receptors are often described as being a lock and key system – only the right key will open the door. The problem with this analogy is that now more is known about receptors, it is more like hand and made-to-measure glove than lock and key. Only the right hand, slipping into the bespoke empty glove, whose fingers trail inside the cell, can fill it correctly in order to set the correct cascade of cell chemicals in motion. Another problem with the lock and key scenario is that it makes it sound as though receptors are permanent fixtures. They aren't. There is something rather Harry Potterish about them: they can suddenly appear in huge quantities or alternatively disappear. Sometimes they can even, alarmingly, become soluble and get dissolved away before the hormone arrives. This means that a certain tissue will suddenly appear to become much more, or less, sensitive to the effects of a hormone, even though the amounts of hormone haven't changed. If you are in a particularly grumpy mood before a period, you may not have that imbalance of hormones so popularly and irritatingly foretold, but rather more receptors than usual. Receptors are not just found on the usual suspect target organs. For instance, you'd expect oestrogen receptors in the ovary and breast, but actually oestrogen receptors are everywhere throughout the body – brain, blood vessels, bone – demonstrating the range of tissues affected by a particular hormone. Almost every week there is an announcement of the finding of a completely unexpected hormone receptor in a particular tissue. What are receptors for the hormone of starvation – leptin – doing in the testes? Or for that matter, growth hormone receptors in breast cancer cells?

There is an exception to the way docking works. Steroid hormones are, unlike the other types of hormone, fat soluble. Cell membranes are made of fat. Steroid hormones don't need surface receptors on the membrane because, being fat soluble, they are able to just melt through the fatty cell membrane like a ghost through a wall, and then use the fatty bits inside the cell as a sort of guide rope route to dock with receptors inside the cells, usually within the nucleus itself.

What Are Hormones Made Of?

Hormones can be divided into three main types. The majority are made of protein – the smaller of these are called peptides – but there are also steroids, made from cholesterol, and finally ones derived from tyrosine which is an amino acid. Amino acids are the building blocks from which all proteins are made.

PROTEINS

Proteins are just chains of amino acids. That's *just* as in '*just* a Leonardo' by the way. A small chain of no more than twenty amino acids is termed a peptide. Over twenty amino acids strung together are called a protein, rather than a peptide (however, this is a bit elastic). The longer the chain, the more likely the protein is to be elaborately folded and shaped. The three-dimensional shape of a protein is crucial to the way it functions. The protein hormones tend to come in tribes, like growth hormone and prolactin, which are almost identical except for a different sequence of amino acids on the end of the chain. Another tribe of big protein hormones include follicle stimulating hormone, luteinising hormone and human chorionic gonadotrophin. They are called glycoproteins, because they also have sugars attached to them. Again, they are very similar, one to another, differing only in one vital section. Although we talk of 'growth hormone' as if it were just one thing, in reality there are a great many natural variants in your body at the same time. It's not known why this happens.

MODIFIED AMINO ACIDS

Another type of hormone uses a specific amino acid – in this case tyrosine – as a sort of generic low loader on to which bespoke carriages are bolted. The hormones that are based on tyrosine include the thyroid hormones and also those called catecholamines, which are produced by the innermost portion of the adrenal glands, and many of which act as neurotransmitters, facilitating messages between nerves. The catecholamines include adrenaline and also noradrenaline which is produced not only in the adrenal gland but also at nerve endings.

STEROIDS

A third category of hormones are steroids. We tend to think of steroids as unpleasant drugs taken by bodybuilders. They are an enormously important group of natural body chemicals, which includes Vitamin D, and the bile acids, which help digestion, as well as the hormones cortisol and aldosterone, produced by the adrenals, and the sex hormones testosterone, progesterone and oestrogen. The basic building block for steroids is cholesterol and by adding different chemical groups to this molecule, completely new and very different substances can be made with, despite their similarity, radically different biological properties.

Steroid production is rather like an assembly line making a Swiss Army knife. You have the basic knife kit (cholesterol) and then various blades get added, so you can have the boy scout version with the knife and horse's hoof cleaner, or the top of the range mountaineer special, with thirty-two blades. The point is that the mountaineer special had to be the boy scout version first – and the steroids are built on the same basis. Another analogy would be with the London Underground. If you take the Piccadilly line, always starting at King's Cross and always finishing at Heathrow, which is the end of the line, you have to go through Holborn and Knightsbridge first. There is no bypass or short cut. It's like that with steroids. The steroid hormone aldosterone which helps control blood pressure has to go through being the reproductive hormone progesterone and the stress hormone cortisol first. The oestrogen oestradiol is made from testosterone (a male hormone), having been oestrone (a female hormone), androstenedione (a male hormone), DHEA (a unisex hormone), and pregnenolone (a female hormone) first.

Steroids, like the tyrosine-derived hormones, seem to be considered a bit of a liability, for they are given chaperones whilst travelling in the blood, called carrier proteins or globulins. Some carriers are specific – sex hormone binding globulin (SHBG) for testosterone, for instance, or thyroid hormone binding globulin

(THBG) – but others are common proteins like albumen, protein tarts who will carry anything – but only loosely bound – and definitely not in the same close heavy armlock as that of the specific binding globulins.

You might have come across the phrase 'free testosterone'. What this means is testosterone that hasn't got a chaperone and isn't locked up by its carrier protein. It's usually the amount of 'free' hormone that determines how well it works. Some endocrine diseases are not caused by having too much or too little of a particular hormone but by changes in the number of chaperones available which effectively either sequesters or releases more 'free' hormone.

What Happens When You Have Too Much or Too Little Hormone

THYROID GLAND

Diseases that are caused by too much or too little hormone are still common. For instance about 700 million people worldwide are estimated to have a goitre, an enlargement of the thyroid gland that is seen as a big lump on the front of the neck. Iodine is essential to the production of the thyroid hormones T_4 and T_3, but many parts of the world, particularly landlocked mountainous areas like the Alps and regions of China, have soil which is deficient in iodine. As a consequence, many people living in iodine-deficient areas have goitre. In Britain, the area around the Peak district was one such affected area and because so many people who lived there had goitre, the condition became known as Derbyshire neck. About 26 million people worldwide have brain damage caused by their thyroid condition, and of these some 6 million are sufficiently mentally handicapped that they are completely dependent on others. This condition is known as cretinism and symptoms include intellectual impairment, hearing or speech problems, stunted growth and poor movement. This misery is caused by the thyroid gland not working as it should because it is unable to obtain the iodine it needs for proper function. It is completely preventable with iodine supplements. In Britain, most of our table salt is now iodized with potassium iodide, and therefore the deficiency is no longer seen.

Thyroid problems can also be made worse by diet. An example is cassava, a staple food in Africa which, if not prepared properly, contains a chemical which blocks uptake of iodine. Soy beans also affect thyroid function, as do vegetables from the cabbage family, like cabbage itself, turnips and broccoli, further reducing what little thyroid hormone there is. The thyroid is rather like an iodine sponge. It will soak up whatever it can get hold of until it can take no more. This is why giving potassium iodide tablets to people in the immediate aftermath of a nuclear explosion will prevent their bodies from taking up radioactive iodine because the thyroid will have been so flooded by iodine that it cannot absorb any more.

Written texts make clear that in the Middle Ages the Chinese knew how to treat goitre and prescribed seaweed (which, like any food from the sea or grown by the sea, contains large quantities of iodine). In the fourteenth century, Chinese physicians recommended treating goitre with fifty desiccated pigs' thyroids, ground up in a glass of wine. Today there is still debate as to whether or not desiccated whole thyroid extract is better than synthetic thyroid hormone.

GROWTH HORMONE

You will also be familiar with the disease caused by lack of insulin – diabetes – and with the conditions caused by too much or too little hormone – dwarfism and gigantism. Growth during the first eight to ten months of life is largely controlled by food intake, but growth hormone then becomes the dominant influence on how children grow. There are also benign balls of cells, tumours, which secrete growth hormone (GH) and this constant production of GH produces as you'd expect, very tall people – seven foot or taller – the condition is known as gigantism. If excess GH is produced after growing has stopped (again because of a tumour), a condition called acromegaly develops, which causes the bones of the hands, feet and jaw to become enlarged.

The First Book of Samuel in the Bible relates the story of David and the giant Goliath, who was said to be six cubits and a span in height. A cubit is an Egyptian measure, roughly the length of the elbow to the tip of the middle finger and reckoned to be eighteen inches. A span is half a cubit, which would make Goliath well over nine foot tall. The tallest man ever recorded was Robert Wadlow, born in Alton, Illinois, in 1918, who was 8′ 11″. He died when he was only twenty-two. Robert Wadlow had a tumour of the pituitary gland in childhood, causing an excess of growth hormone. Did Goliath have a hormone problem? I doubt it. Too much growth hormone does not make you a muscle-bound superman as we'll see in later chapters. Quite the reverse is usually the case, with respiratory problems, diabetes and high blood pressure being the norm and disabling osteoarthritis of load-bearing joints also an early feature. By his teens, Robert Wadlow needed a walking stick.

Another common problem for those subjected to too much growth hormone is carpal tunnel syndrome, which is caused by pressure on the median nerve in the wrists, and results in numbness and loss of power in the hands. This would have made it impossible for Goliath to hold heavy items like his staff, which the Bible tells us 'was like a weaver's beam', let alone his spear, of which the head alone 'weighed six hundred shekels of iron'.

Although a very rare form of acromegaly is inherited, most cases are caused by malfunctions of the pituitary and so are 'one offs'. A further hint on Goliath's physique comes from the Second Book of Samuel in which it is noted that four more giants had been killed in battle by the Israelites. All are said to come from the tribe of Gath. This sounds as if the Gathites were just exceedingly tall and six cubits and a span is a myth.

However, the opposite case has been made persuasively by endocrinologist Shlomo Melmed of the Cedars Sinai Medical Center, Los Angeles. He argues that Goliath's height was definitely the result of a pituitary tumour arising in childhood. Such tumours often press upon the optic nerve, leading to loss of peripheral vision, which might account for his seeming unawareness of David and his sling. A blow to the head for a person with this condition could have caused a massive haemorrhage, leading to death, even from a seemingly minor head injury.

The point of the story is surely that David was small by comparison and won the fight through applied weapons technology (a well-aimed sling-shot). A rather more likely sufferer from acromegaly was the Egyptian pharaoah Akhenaten, whose portraits show the typical projecting jaw of the condition.

ADRENAL GLANDS

John F. Kennedy suffered from Addison's disease, in which the cortex of the adrenal glands atrophies, resulting in life-threatening deficiencies of cortisol and aldosterone. Up until 1940, Addison's disease was invariably fatal, but it was then discovered that it could be treated with cortisone. Kennedy was diagnosed by a London doctor in 1947, at a time when cortisone was an extremely expensive drug: the Kennedys were said to keep quantities of the drug in safety deposit boxes around the world. Had Kennedy not been a rich man, he would not have survived, because cheaper, synthetic versions of cortisone weren't widely available until the 1950s. As it was, he was so ill that after the diagnosis he was told that he had only a year to live and was actually given the last rites on his return sea voyage to the States.

Kennedy also suffered from serious back problems and was in so much pain that in 1954, when he was a US Senator, surgery became necessary. This can be an extremely hazardous undertaking in someone with Addison's disease. He pulled through, but with many complications, and repeat surgery was needed. So unusual was his survival that it was written up as an anonymous case report in the *Journal of the American Medical Association* in 1955. No one knew that '37-year-old male' was in fact John F. Kennedy until 1967, four years after his death. He also looked much healthier than he was because, ironically, another feature of Addison's disease is a bronzing of the skin caused by abnormal synthesis of melanin pigment in the skin.

When he was standing for President in 1960, his campaign team flatly denied that he had Addison's disease. They relied on a very narrow definition of Addison's as a disease only caused by tuberculosis of the adrenals, to quash rumours of ill-health. Tuberculosis was about the only disease Kennedy didn't have. Like Franklin D. Roosevelt before him, Kennedy managed to overcome debilitating health problems to become one of America's greatest presidents.

The novelist Jane Austen, on the other hand, almost certainly did have TB-induced Addison's disease. In an article in the *British Medical Journal* in July 1964, Sir Zachary Cope pointed out that Jane Austen had herself identified a key feature of the disease in a letter to her brother of 23 March 1817: 'Recovering my looks a little, which have been bad enough, black and white and every wrong colour.' 'There is no disease', wrote Sir Zachary, 'other than Addison's disease that could present a face that was "black and white" and at the same time give rise to the other symptoms described in her letters.'

You can do without ovaries, thyroid, pancreas – in fact most endocrine organs – provided that you receive the appropriate hormone supplements. But there is one exception. Remove both adrenal glands and you will die very quickly. There is no substitute, no way of mimicking the extraordinary second-by-second adjustments that the stress hormones of the adrenal glands make to crucial body functions. Without these glands, there is no recovery from physical or emotional trauma, no proper control of blood pressure, water balance or heart rate.

Complete loss of an endocrine gland is an extreme cause of

having too little of a hormone. There are many other causes of deficiency – or excess. As we have seen, there are many steps involved in the production of a hormone, so insufficiency is not simply about not having enough of the hormone itself. Faults in any part of the chain might be the problem: in the hypothalamus, by there not being enough releasing hormone; in the pituitary, by failure of its hormones; by faulty production in the site of hormone manufacture; by poorly functioning or absent receptors or failure of the feedback systems, and so on, right down the chain.

Almost Hormones

As research has moved on, the definition of hormones has had to become rather elastic. Many of the newly discovered hormones affect cells around them, or even the cell that produced them. The discovery of other chemicals in the body has made the scientific community realize that many other molecules have jobs as chemical messengers and regulators, and that the hormone club is not quite as exclusive as originally thought. Here are three of the principal contenders for quasi-hormone status.

PROSTAGLANDINS

Amino acids are used to build the peptides and proteins of many hormones, whereas cholesterol is the building block of steroids. Another basic material is fatty acid, the major storage component of fat. Fatty acids are used to manufacture a type of strictly local hormone called a prostaglandin. The first prostaglandin that was isolated was found in semen and was thought to have been secreted by the prostate gland, hence the name. It is now known that almost all tissues produce prostaglandins, which act locally. Prosta-glandins are strictly local in their action, and also have a regulatory role.

Prostaglandins get involved in all sorts of bodily reactions such as muscle contraction and inflammation, and are familiar to women in their role in period pain. The reason why aspirin works so well for period pain is because it's an anti-prostaglandin. Prostaglandins are sometimes called 'hormone-like', sometimes 'pre-hormones', and many endocrinologists are now calling them hormones.

CYTOKINES

The endocrine system doesn't work in isolation but in concert with other systems of the body. It has a particularly close relationship with the immune system. Cytokines are molecules secreted by immune cells that can regulate the endocrine system. There are many, many cytokines, some of whose names are familiar, like interferons, given as a treatment to those with multiple sclerosis. Another large, less familiar class of cytokines are interleukins. When you are seriously injured – a severe burn for instance – levels of stress hormones, especially cortisol and adrenaline, soar. From what you have read so far, you would think that this must be organized through the hypothalamus, which dispatches corticotrophin releasing hormone to the anterior pituitary, which then sends out adrenocorticotrophin to the adrenal cortex, which then responds by a rapid increase in stress hormones. In fact it doesn't work like this in serious trauma because cytokines bypass the normal routes, taking messages direct to the adrenal glands themselves. In a sense, cytokines are acting in the same way as adrenocorticotrophin – even though they are not hormones.

NITRIC OXIDE

You will know nitric oxide (NO) better as a gas – it's a major component of exhaust fumes and smog and was generally thought to be A Bad Thing – a poisonous asthma-inducing pollutant. Indeed, caution has been advised ever since Sir Humphrey Davy was nearly killed in 1800 when he decided to see what would happen when he inhaled it. Yet in the 1980s the very same molecule was discovered to be vital to the health of both body and mind – and to have a distinctly hormone-like action, as a locally produced messenger and regulator. The story of nitric acid started when it was discovered in 1867 that amyl nitrite (most familiar as the recreational drug, 'poppers') could relieve both high blood pressure and angina pain. Sir Arthur Conan Doyle, who was a GP in Southsea, certainly knew about it, for in the Sherlock Holmes story, 'The Case of the Resident Patient', written in 1893, 'amyl of nitrite' is mentioned as a treatment for lowering the blood pressure of a man affected by catalepsy. Its use for lowering blood pressure had been prompted by a chemist reporting flushing of his face and heart pounding during an experiment with amyl nitrite.

Something very similar had also occurred in munitions workers. The explosive nitroglycerine had been discovered in 1846. Commercial production had been pioneered by Alfred Nobel in Sweden, but it was highly unstable. He discovered how to reduce its sensitivity to shock, producing dynamite and making a fortune in the process, which he used to fund the Nobel prizes. Munitions workers handling explosives also had very low blood pressure, together with flushed hands and faces. In an extraordinary leap of faith, nitroglycerine was placed under the tongue in an attempt to provide a more long-lasting relief of pain for angina than amyl nitrite. The treatment worked and nitroglycerine is still the treatment of choice for angina pain.

For a century, no one knew why it worked so well. What links these seemingly disparate pieces of information is nitric oxide. It is released from both amyl nitrite and nitroglycerine and controls the muscle tone of blood vessel walls, dilating them and easing pain and blood pressure. This wasn't discovered until 1987 by Salvador Moncada. It is now known that nitric oxide is an essential part of the physiology of most organs and tissues, including the brain, where it is linked to memory formation. The erection of the penis, for instance, is mediated by nitric oxide released from nerve endings close to the blood vessels of the penis – Viagra works by enhancing this effect. That is why taking amyl nitrite *and* Viagra is a recipe for disaster because too much nitric oxide is produced, and the result is usually a heart attack. It is a stiffy not a stiff that is required.

Nitric oxide affects secretion from several endocrine glands, including gonadotrophin releasing hormone from the hypothalamus and adrenaline from the adrenals. It regulates, it stimulates production of a hormone – and sounds pretty much like a hormone. However, it falls just beyond the scope of this book and so that is the last you will hear of this ubiquitous and intriguing molecule here.

Let me now start filling in the detail as I go on to describe the wonderful elegance of the hormonal system – as it relates to love, attraction and sex.

CHAPTER TWO

HORMONE EXPLOSIONS 1
Attraction, Sex and Babies

Attraction

People in the West may pour scorn on the whole notion of arranged marriages, preferring the romantic ideal of marrying for love, rather than for money or for strategic alliances. Meanwhile, their hormones are busily brokering marriages behind the scenes. Free will? I don't think so, madam. We're talking sexual chemistry here, with your brain playing Cupid, and your hormones providing the arrows.

So you walk into a crowded room and there he is. Your heart pounds, your stomach churns and your face suddenly blushes crimson. You may want to play it cool, but your body is gearing itself up for action, lots of it. Your body is dosing itself with adrenaline, sending signals to places that are good at losing heat, like your cheeks. You turn away, hoping he hasn't seen you. But he has. You have big breasts and a relatively narrow waist, which are tonight seductively enclosed in a new dress. Your hormones are advertising their wares, for these body proportions are linked with up to 40 per cent higher levels of female hormones mid-cycle, making it highly likely that you are very fertile. Subconsciously that message is received by his brain. The rush of testosterone is sufficient to alter his behaviour and his mood. He wants you.

You sneak a look at his face. Shaped by testosterone in the womb, his jawline is strong and masculine, which is attractive to you, particularly since you are close to ovulation, when women have the greatest preference for masculine features. Had he much stronger features, indicating higher levels of testosterone, it would have been a turn-off to you, for too much testosterone is associated with negative personality traits, such as aggression and infidelity. He comes over.

'It's hot in here – let's go out on the verandah,' he says. He is very close. You're conscious of his body and how it smells. Enticing. He takes you in his arms and kisses you. You are conscious of dampness between your legs. Yes, your hormones are telling you, this could be the one. Meanwhile his hormones are sending the same messages about you.

Hormones and sex are intimately entwined. Encouraging and enabling, they are responsible for ensuring that our species continues. This chapter is the truth about hormones, love and sex.

Smell is one of the senses carrying information about the outside environment back to the brain. We tend to regard smell as the least important of the five senses in humans, and in fact our olfactory lobes are tiny compared to those of most other mammals. Yet we all know that smell can be the most powerfully evocative of our senses, transporting us back to times past. The smell of hot sun on wood takes me instantly to a beach hut that we used as children, flooding my brain with memories of sandy sandwiches. We are aware, too, that smell can be life-saving – for instance, in detecting the smell of gas. Smell also directs behaviour too. The reek of spoiled and rotting food triggers feelings of disgust so that we reject foodstuffs that are likely to be harmful, spitting them out or vomiting.

The nose and sexuality are equally powerfully linked and it is hormones that provide the go-between. A quick sniff of the female rear, perhaps coupled with a tentative tasting, is a central part of male mammal behaviour, for it immediately tells the male whether the female is on heat or not. Male rhesus monkeys certainly recognize the reproductive status of females in this way, reserving maximum frequency of ejaculation for females in oestrus. By contrast, human females are much more coy, and do not obviously broadcast information about their cycle, indeed many women don't even know themselves whether or not they are ovulating. Most women would feel uncomfortable if they thought that a man could detect the stage of their cycle from their smell, especially if menstrual blood could be smelt from afar. All that most women would like men to know from their smell is that they wash often and use Chanel No. 5.

Yet every woman has a signature smell – their very own personal perfume. It is presumed that the Bartholin's glands, either side of the vaginal opening, which secrete a clear alkaline fluid during sexual arousal, are the source of this alluring scent. These glands are under the control of ovarian hormones. So do men sense what we women might guess at, but can't know for sure, just from our smell?

There is some evidence that they do. Men exposed to synthetic vaginal secretions at various stages of the menstrual cycle find them unpleasant. However, if they are asked to sniff them while looking at pictures of attractive women, they report them as more attractive. In addition, simulated ovulation scents send their testosterone levels soaring. Almost certainly, if you asked men to tell you whether the women in their lives were ovulating, they wouldn't have a clue. Yet unconsciously their bodies know and respond physiologically with increases in testosterone.

Hormones certainly alter women's sense of smell at key points in their lives. For instance, pregnant women report having a 'stuffed-up nose' feeling during pregnancy. This is because nasal membranes become swollen in response to increased amounts of blood oestrogens. They are also much more sensitive to smell – it's a common phenomenon for women to become acutely sensitized to one particular smell in pregnancy. I developed a loathing for Lux soap, which suddenly I could detect a mile away, even if wrapped. Conversely, smell is lessened in women at menopause when oestrogen levels drop. Pre-menopausal women report heightened smell sensations and nose stuffiness at the time of ovulation.

Why should women be more sensitive to smell at ovulation? The reason it could be important was revealed by intriguing research from a team in Bern, Switzerland, in 1995. The major histocompatibility complex (MHC) is the section of your DNA that carries instructions for a key part of your immune system, which is your body's defence system. It is highly variable. It appears that the MHC complex influences both body odours and body odour preferences. In women, this preference depends on their hormonal status. In a classic experiment, female and male students were typed for certain genes within their MHC complex. Each male student wore a Y-shirt for two consecutive nights and the girls were then asked to rate the smell of each shirt. The women most liked the smells of men whose MHC differed from their own and least liked those from men whose MHC was most similar to their own. Significantly, the 'alike' smells also reminded them most of former partners. This difference in odour assessment was reversed if the women were taking oral contraceptives (which suppresses ovulation). Thus only if women were ovulating was there a specific mate preference based on smell in which men of a particular genetic type were preferred.

It has been suggested that there is an evolutionary advantage in choosing a mate with a different MHC from your own. The more genetic cards you have to shuffle with, the more likely you are to create an MHC gene variant in your offspring that can outfox and be able to resist parasites – a major consideration in our past. There is also evidence that the pregnancies of couples whose MHCs are very similar are more likely to end in miscarriage, probably because a baby with a similar MHC to its mother doesn't switch off the mother's immune response as effectively as it should. This leads to a recognition of the baby as 'foreign' and its rejection.

There are actually some very subtle visual clues as well: for instance, women's faces become more symmetrical around the time of ovulation. Symmetricality is an attribute that human beings seem to prize. Take a picture of a woman, divide it in half and recompose the photo, so that one side of the face is a mirror image of the other. Now ask people to say which is more attractive, the before or after picture? They consistently pick the 'after' picture and strongly associate symmetry with attractiveness.

These clues, provided by scent and sight, are worthless unless the brain is able to translate the signals, decide on a course of action (make a move on this man now) and effect a change in behaviour or physiology. And hormones are key to this, particularly the neuro-endocrine system, in which hormones alter behaviour or mood through an effect on the brain. The proof of the pudding would be if sexual frequency and orgasm were to increase when women ovulate, thus making them want sex at a time when they are most likely to conceive. There have been a large number of studies in this area, but they produce conflicting results. Much of the methodology has been suspect, including self-reporting of arousal and ovulation in some studies. The consensus seems to be that women report increased levels of desire in the latter part of the early (follicular) stage of their cycle, but they do so again just before their period.

Research from Steven Gangestad and others from the University of New Mexico found that women reported greater interest and fantasy about men other than their long-term partners near ovulation, though this effect was not noted in their partner. Interestingly, the partner himself was more attentive and proprietorial closer to ovulation. If this is a genuine effect, then it must be hormone-mediated, and unconscious – because, as we have noted, most men wouldn't know whether their partner was ovulating (most men wouldn't know what their partner was wearing, let alone ovulating).

There has been relatively little work relating to dreams and the menstrual cycle, but what there is seems to suggest that erotic dreams are most likely to be experienced by women at times when they feel least sexual when awake – for instance, during their periods. Orgasm does not appear to be more frequent at ovulation. But it is very difficult to disentangle physiology from the overlay of life's rich pattern. A delayed journey, tiredness and a pile of ironing, and your hormones can go whistle.

So having established that you are the one for him, how do you bond? Studies of prairie voles have revealed the role of two hormones in romance. Oxytocin is the hormone of breastfeeding, but is also called the cuddling hormone. Vasopressin has been called 'the monogamy hormone'. In prairie voles, mating is the prelude to pair bonding and if male voles are given a drug that stops vasopressin from working, the vole fails to be smitten by his volette. Nor does he actively pursue potential love rivals as he would have done when spurred on by vasopressin. If given more vasopressin, attachment is strengthened. Humans also secrete oxytocin and vasopressin at the appropriate moment. Oxytocin is released when you look at the one you love. Hormones are now being deployed in a concerted attempt to get you to stay together, long enough not only to have a baby but also to nurture it to independence.

Sex

Part of the pleasure in sex for women is the experience within her vagina, whose elasticity and thickness are maintained by oestrogen. After the menopause, a thinning drying vagina can be a bar to sexual enjoyment. Orgasm, however, is maintained by another hormone altogether.

When a women has an orgasm, her womb contracts. Intrauterine pressures increase, as does vaginal pressure. When orgasm is over, the intrauterine pressure drops very rapidly, creating a pressure gradient. The cervix dips and then, thanks to that pressure gradient, literally hoovers sperm into the womb. Orgasm isn't strictly necessary to conception, but it is designed to make the most of your chances. Oxytocin is the hormone at work here. It is thought of as the hormone of birth. Indeed, the word oxytocin comes from the Greek for 'quick birth' and under its influence the womb – which is made of smooth muscle – contracts rhythmically and powerfully to expel the baby. Almost all of a woman's genital apparatus is made of smooth muscle (which is under involuntary control, unlike the striped muscles of, say, your biceps). Oxytocin is responsible for the dilation of your pupils as you orgasm, the gaping of the cervix into a round 'O' (which, incidentally, is mirrored in the shape of your mouth during orgasm) and the rhythmic contractions of orgasm. The greater the amount of oxytocin, the more intense the orgasm. And the better the orgasm, the more oxytocin is knocking about to ensure that you bond with the man that thought he, rather than your hormones, was responsible for your pleasure. So is this surge of oxytocin all about your pleasure? No. The point of the contractions is to ensure egg and sperm transport. The contraction is so exquisitely directed that the human female is capable, if necessary, of organizing egg and sperm movement in opposite directions at the same time.

In the mid-1990s zoologist and evolutionary biologist Dr Robin Baker claimed that women were effectively able to sort sperm in utero, actively choosing that ejaculate which was most favourable from amongst multiple partners. Lest that in itself sounds improbable, a Britsh sex survey of the 1980s revealed that over 70 per cent of women had during their lifetime slept with two men within the space of five days; nearly 70 per cent had done so within a day of each other and 1 per cent claimed to have done so within thirty minutes. Despite taking these surveys with a pinch of salt – how many of us have filled in the 'five times a night' box during a boring lunch hour spent with our mates, only for it to be taken at face value by an unquestioning academic – there is evidence throughout the animal world of active sperm-sorting. Hamsters, for instance, are very selective about sperm, allowing only a few of the millions deposited through. Nevertheless fertilization rates are close to 100 per cent. Female mice are able to recognize which sperm are more compatible – in terms of compatible MHCs – and sperm that are deemed a bad match are left behind. Polyandry – multiple mating – is the norm in many animals and a capacity for active vaginal sorting allows the fittest sperm to be selected for fast-track access to the ovum.

Robin Baker outlines his theories on the subject in his book *Sperm Wars*. His ideas are intriguing, although it has to be said, in humans at least, distinctly light on proof. But the sorting mechanisms he proposes depend on muscle movement initiated by oxytocin. However, recent work from the University of Memphis, published in the journal *Nature*, has strengthened the concept of sperm competition, revealing that there is an increase in the amount of sperm in the ejaculate of meadow voles able to smell rival suitors in the air, when pursuing their volette.

It is often assumed that male sexual performance is dictated by testosterone and that if men have erection problems, it is all down to a lack of testosterone. As far as sex is concerned, testosterone is the hormone of sex drive and desire, rather than the hormone which controls function of the penis. It is rather unusual for erectile dysfunction to be caused by a hormone problem. Difficulties with erections are more likely to be caused by faults in the exquisitely designed hydraulic system on which a rampant penis depends. The mechanics of it are dictated by blood flow and it is alterations in blood flow caused by narrowed arteries, diabetes, prescription drugs, drinking or smoking that are the principal cause of dysfunction. In fact, there is nothing more frustrating to a man than having all his hormones in full flood, goading him on, only to discover that he has a non-playing member on the team. Poor levels of testosterone in men are in fact not a normal cause of impotence. This has not stopped – as you will discover in the penultimate chapter of this book – charlatans recommending testosterone to ageing men as the certain way to eternity and grateful women.

Lack of testosterone may, in fact, be more of a problem in women in terms of sexual dysfunction. The tissue of women's genitals are androgen-dependent, including the pubic hair and nipples as well as the labia and clitoris. You will recall that the adrenals churn out androgens – male hormones – in both men and women.

The ovaries also produce testosterone: some is manufactured start to finish, as it were, but about half of it is made from semi-assembled raw material, supplied in the form of the androgen DHEA, produced by the adrenals. In fact, the most abundant sex hormone in women's circulation is not oestrogen but the androgen DHEA, or, to be strictly accurate, its sulphated form DHEAS. One of the functions of DHEAS is as a semi-finished construction material, handy for conversion into testosterone in sites like hair follicles, but it is also important as a construction material for oestrogen production.

As women age, levels of testosterone fall, by roughly half from twenty to forty years of age. This is not simply because of decreasing amounts of testosterone being produced, but because of an increase in the amount of those steroid chaperones, SHBGs, which lock up more of what is being produced and make even less 'free' testosterone available. There has been an attempt of late to medicalize sex problems in women. The manufacturers of testosterone implants would have us believe that 40 per cent of women have sexual dysfunction requiring medical treatment. There are certainly physiological problems that affect women's desire and arousal, just as there are in men, such as decreased blood flow through poor general health and prescription drugs (especially the pill, Valium and some of the SSRIs (Selective Serotonin Reuptake Inhibitors) used for depression). Such problems are no doubt greatly under-reported and when they are, are not dealt with all that sympathetically.

However, whether the testosterone fall with age is responsible for declining sexual activity in women is a moot point. Researchers at the Jean Hailes Foundation in Australia, who tracked changing hormone levels with age in a large group of women as part of the Sue Ismiel International Study into Women's Health and Hormones, found that low testosterone levels bore no significant relationship to low libido in women from age eighteen right up to seventy-five. But they did find that a low DHEA level made it three times more likely that there would be poor sexual function –

remember, DHEA is made into both testosterone and oestrogen.

Sex has never just been about physiology. There is a strong psychological factor too and the belief that a pill, testosterone, DHEA or whatever could magically conjure desire and arousal when all you have at home is a boring, overweight smelly bloke whose idea of foreplay is to say 'turn over, it's your lucky night' is unlikely to say the least. Having said all of that, testosterone implants and patches are claimed to have a genuine and enduring effect on women with sexual dysfunction, particularly those who are said to suffer from FADS, Female Androgen Deficiency Syndrome. Lack of desire might well be down to hormones – in which case it's worth checking it out, particularly if there has previously been no problem. But it can also be BWB syndrome (as in Bored with Bloke). There is no dispute about testosterone replacement in women who have had their ovaries removed completely before the menopause, and the inclusion of testosterone as part of their hormone replacement regimen is now considered important, particularly in maintaining libido.

Finally, science occasionally throws up those 'no, never' types of study. One, which received a great deal of publicity, was the Archives of Sexual Behaviour study, published in 2002, from a team at the State University of New York, which concluded that semen makes you happy. It compared women whose partners wore condoms, with women whose partners did not. Those who did use condoms were more depressed (their mood was assessed using a standard mood questionnaire called the Beck Depression Inventory). The time interval since their last protected encounter made no difference to their general misery. The non-condom users, on the other hand, were less depressed but the longer the interval since their last sexual encounter the worse their mood. The researchers concluded that this illustrated hormones at work – being absorbed from semen through the vaginal mucosa. Semen does indeed contain a cocktail of hormones, including, as you might imagine, testosterone, but also oestrogens, prolactin and a clutch of prostaglandins. However, there is somewhere between 8 and 80 picogrammes of oestradiol per millilitre of semen – which is a tiny amount.

This is the kind of research that scores a direct hit on your common-sense gene, and makes you say 'yes, but what about …'. Perhaps women who used condoms were of a different personality type, or the ones who didn't had more stable, sexually fulfilling relationships which made them happier. The researchers said that none of these factors could explain their findings. They claimed, less than convincingly, that men who made women feel happy were likely to have more chances to impregnate them, which would be biologically advantageous. Does this mean, since some steroid hormones survive the digestion process, that oral sex is mood-enhancing? Hmm. I wouldn't count on it being on prescription as a replacement for Prozac in the near future. To be bold about this, you'd have to ship an awful lot of semen on board for it to make any real difference to your hormone levels. The andrologists that I consulted were unanimous. You get more oestrogen from one contraceptive pill than you would from – and their estimates varied – at least forty-three separate inseminations, assuming 5–12 ml per shot. Given that most (young) men can only run to half a dozen emissions a day, before temporarily running dry, you might want to find an alternative form of happiness therapy.

Conception

The sex of your child is determined by its chromosomes. If a baby has XX, she's a girl, XY and he's a boy. Eggs and sperm are the only cells in the body that have half a set of chromosomes (haploid, if you want to be technical). All eggs provide an X, but each sperm provides either an X or a Y. Effectively sperm dictate gender. So it's all down to chromosomes then – and utterly random? No. Sex is decided by hormones on several counts.

In theory, you have the same 50:50 chance of conceiving a girl or a boy at each act of intercourse. There's good evidence that sex ratios vary according to conditions and even the occupation of the father. Babies conceived in the spring are more likely to be boys, as are those conceived during wartime. Male conceptions are more likely at the beginning or end of the fertile period around ovulation, whereas female conceptions are more likely in the middle. Frequent sex is associated with male offspring, with the effect noted in horses, rats, mice and seals as well as humans.

Unusual offspring sex ratios are associated with a number of specific obstetric conditions. Boys are more common with placenta praevia, a condition in which the placenta lies across the bottom of the womb, blocking the baby's exit; girls with hyperemesis gravidarum (that's when sickness in pregnancy becomes overwhelming). Illness too seems to dictate sex ratios – hepatitis B carriers have more sons. Men destined to suffer (and those diagnosed with) testicular cancer have an excess of girls. Then there is parental occupation. Abalone fishers (an abalone is a highly prized Australian mollusc that lives in deep water) and other divers have more daughters as do professional drivers, pilots of high-performance aircraft, anaesthetists and astronauts.

So what's this all about? The theory – advanced in particular by Dr William James of the Galton Laboratory at University College London – is that it's parental hormone levels around the time of conception that make the difference. High concentrations of testosterone and oestrogen increase the chances of having a son, high concentrations of progesterone and luteinising hormone favour girls.

Now let's look at those sex ratio anomalies again. Testosterone is reduced in divers and abalone fishers, probably in response to a pressure stress while in deep water. They have more girls, as do astronauts, who, perhaps surprisingly, are claimed to have low testosterone levels. Those with testicular cancer have low testosterone levels, whereas hepatitis B carriers have high levels and this is reflected by their offspring. Chronic hardship, such as that experienced in wars or epidemics, appears to raise testosterone levels in women, thus temporarily raising the number of women suited to conceiving male offspring. Frequent sex – which presumably occurs during spring when the sap is rising and also soon after marriage – favours boys. In fact, the greater likelihood of a boy as a first born is attributed to the honeymoon effect. Conception in the middle of your cycle, when luteinising hormone is at its greatest, tends to beget girls.

There are many other anomalies to consider. Presidents and prime ministers tend to have an excess of girls. The theory here is that men who are seriously stressed, as presumably presidents are – have high levels of stress hormones, which depress levels of testosterone (in women, stress raises testosterone). Your average unstressed alpha male begets boys.

The general rule is that more testosterone in women produces boys; less testosterone in men produces girls. This is fascinating stuff, although some of the data is a bit thin, and if you're mad to have a girl, I wouldn't go rushing out to find an abalone fisherman on the strength of this work.

But there's much more. The so-called Trivers and Willard hypothesis, published some thirty years ago in the journal *Science* – is that reproductive success should be greater in parents who can manipulate the sex of their offspring according to their own condition. If times are relatively hard – a drought, lack of food for instance – daughters are favoured, while when times are good, there is an investment in sons. The reasoning is that daughters, even those not in tip-top shape, will probably still get pregnant. But sons are a different matter. Their reproductive success is far from assured, so, if you want to guarantee as many descendants as you can, being able to produce girls in hard times is a better strategy. There's much work that backs this up too in animal populations, such as caribou (the animals that Trivers and Willard studied). We can see that such an effect might be important in marmosets or moose, but humans? Aren't we above that sort of thing? More in control of our own destinies? It appears not.

There have been many studies on humans which support this theory, including most recently work from the Biological Anthropology Research Group at the University of Kent, which showed that there is an association between the sex of a woman's first child and the age the mother believes she might reach. When two groups of women, one affluent, one deprived, were asked how long they thought they each would live, the women who were well resourced and healthy, or even those that were poor but happy with their lot, expected to live longer than those who were not. It's called the subjective life expectancy. And indeed, women who were optimists and believed that they would reach a ripe old age were more likely to have had a son as their first born.

Here you have social environment and perceived physical conditions influencing testosterone levels and the gender of offspring, all linked and orchestrated by the hormones. It's extraordinary.

The Trivers and Willard hypothesis doesn't always hold true. Times were hard during and after the Second World War, yet war conditions irrefutably result in more boys, not girls. Some scientists, notably Dr Valerie Grant, of the University of Auckland, believe that it's less about 'condition' and more about dominance, a biological determinant that is underpinned by testosterone. So here we are, back with hormones again. This idea – the maternal dominance theory – says that the females who are most dominant (who would presumably have a greater share of resources) are the ones who have boys, whilst the less successful ones have girls. A dominant woman – and here we mean a woman who is successful in life – is likely to have higher circulating levels of testosterone, and to produce boys rather than girls. Indeed, an analysis by Grant of 353 women who were sufficiently high-achieving to have entries in a national dictionary of biography revealed a significantly high ratio of boys to girls among their children.

The mechanics of how this all happens is anyone's guess. It might be that Y-bearing sperm get an open run at the egg, perhaps because conditions in the fallopian tube are adjusted to suit them, or that the lining of the womb is more picky than we will ever know about fertilized eggs, rejecting not just those that are sub-standard but those of the 'wrong' sex too. Or it might be that the egg itself can be programmed to reject X-bearing sperm in favour of Y ones. It could all be in the timing, with a conception delay into the 'right' phase of the cycle. However, every single one of these options would need to be mediated by hormonal messaging from the mother.

It's not just internal levels of hormone that determine gender. An unusual sex ratio of births amongst children born to parents of a particular occupation tends to ring alarm bells as to the toxicity of their environment. For instance, in the 1980s far more girl babies than normal were born to American dads who were carbon setters, a dirty job carried out in a type of aluminium reduction plant which is now obsolete.

A study of butchers was also revealing. A letter was published in *The Lancet* (7 March 1987) which reviewed the birth sex ratios of butchers and meat-cutters, who not surprisingly eat more meat than most of us. In 1931, butchers had the usual 50:50 girls to boys sex ratio. But by 1978 the sex ratio had altered and butchers had more girls than boys. In the early 1980s, it had changed again, with an excess of boys. The authors, a team at Ninewells Medical School, Dundee, attributed the first change to the use of oestrogens in meat, but the second to the increasing switch to androgens in meat production in the late 1970s.

The fact that this is happening shouldn't surprise us. Remember that hormones communicate an instruction to do something because of a changed condition on the outside. Our bodies are still making their own decisions about what's good for us individually and as a species. Hormones are the slaves that make it happen.

Pregnancy

Pregnancy is hormone-driven and hormone-maintained; birth is hormone-initiated, as is lactation. Having a baby means that for the best part of a year, hormones are in complete control of your life and that of your baby. So it's hardly surprising that women complain that they feel 'hormonal' during pregnancy. Their bodies are exposed to industrial levels of steroids, principally oestrogen and progesterone. Women on average experience a peak progesterone level of 30 mg per twenty-four hours during their menstrual cycles. During pregnancy, that rises to 75 mg per twenty-four hours at twenty weeks and a walloping 300 mg by forty weeks. Oestrogen levels soar not just tenfold but a hundredfold. One of the oestrogens – oestradiol – increases a thousandfold. This tidal wave of hormones also engulfs the baby.

Progesterone is such a strong sedative that, in high doses, it can be used as an anaesthetic. In fact, its action in the brain is just like that of barbiturates. It may help explain why women feel so cowlike, particularly in late pregnancy. Some scientists believe it may also be an amnesiac. They argue that if amnesia were not associated with childbirth, would any woman ever embark on another pregnancy, if they had clear recall of the pain involved in giving birth?

The influence of hormones turns the inside of the womb from parquet floor to luxurious shag pile and back again within each cycle. The purpose of the shag pile is to provide a welcome mat for a fertilized egg, in which it will be able to embed. If it does embed, an elegantly beautiful hormone sequence is triggered. The dominant follicle, which developed an egg within it and which won the race to release *the* egg that month, is a crumpled remnant of its former self. It's called a corpus luteum (meaning yellow body) and it still has a vital role. It produces just enough progesterone and oestrogen to ensure that the lining is maintained in tip-top luxuriousness. Meanwhile, from about day 14 after conception (likely to be the day you miss your period) the surface bit of the fertilized egg sac that forms the outer surface of the placenta (the chorion) starts to secrete a hormone called chorionic gonadotrophin (hCG), which is almost identical to luteinising hormone except for one teeny section – the beta chain. HCG assumes control of the spent follicle, the corpus luteum, and signals a 'no more LH thanks' message back to the pituitary. This means ovulation is switched off for the time being.

The presence of hCG in the urine is the basis of pregnancy tests. Today, you can buy pregnancy test kits at any chemist. They are simple to use, accurate and the results are available within ten minutes. Essentially the tests use a sniffer dog approach, and search for that little beta chain section of hCG. It is astonishing to realize that until the mid-1960s, pregnancy was confirmed using toads. The South African clawed toad (*Xenopus laevis*) was the toad of choice. It has, as its name suggests, big claws on its rear legs. To be honest, although it looks like a toad, it is actually a frog.

The celebrated zoologist Lancelot Hogben discovered that hGC, the hormone of human pregnancy, was also the hormone that makes female frogs lay eggs. Hogben was determined to use *Xenopus* as a reliable bioassay. The idea was that if urine injected into the frog contained hCG, then within 8–12 hours it would start to lay eggs. But there were many problems. The frogs had to be kept in warm and well-lit conditions or they wouldn't perform. There was also a long-running and tedious dispute with another group of scientists about who did what first, exacerbated when the procedure was named the 'Hogben test'. In 1937, the Edinburgh labs imported 1,500 frogs direct from South Africa and quickly decided that the Hogben test was easily the quickest and best pregnancy test. Many other laboratories acquired their own populations of *Xenopus*. After the Second World War, frog hormone oracles were even available for consultation in Sloane Street, in the basement of the Family Planning Association Clinic. And *Xenopus* carried on providing discerning pregnancy testing until the mid-1960s, when, thank goodness, it was made redundant by newly emerging chemical testing.

Three Months Gone

Under the influence of this pregnancy indicating hormone hCG, the corpus luteum continues to grow and secrete steroids. By twelve weeks, hCG has reached its peak and it then declines, along with the corpus luteum. By this time, it has done its work, for the placenta is now sufficiently developed to be pumping out its own steroids, which begin to rise very rapidly around this time.

The placenta produces a whole raft of hormones and is now considered to be an endocrine gland in its own right. Among the more important hormones are progesterone, several flavours of oestrogen, cortisol and something called human placental lactogen, whose function is not entirely clear. It is probably to do with fetal growth and hCG. Progesterone raises temperature – which is why pregnant women feel like human radiators – it increases fat storage, stops the gut emptying so quickly, and increases gut water resorption to such an extent that constipation may occur. It pumps up the breasts and, to cap it all, may be the hormone responsible for inducing nausea. Oestrogens too pour off the placental production line and control the growth of the womb and its function, as well as the breasts. They make the connective tissue more pliable so that the cervix and pelvis will stretch when the time comes to give birth and are also responsible for the shiny thick hair that women acquire when pregnant. A note on another astonishing thing that happens: if you stretch a muscle, it will want to contract back again, a bit like an elastic band, and yet the womb – which is nothing but a thumping great bag of muscle – is stretched to kingdom come by a growing baby and yet it doesn't contract until it is time for it to do so. That's the wonder of hormones for you.

Another extraordinary aspect of pregnancy is the way that the baby helps manufacture the steroids which will flood the mother's blood supply. The daily steroid production of an unstressed adult is 35 mg per day. Compare this with what the baby produces near term – 200 mg a day. A fall-off in this production rate is sometimes the first hint that the baby is not in good health, which is why measuring the amount of one of these steroids, oestriol, in the mother's urine is a useful test of fetal well-being.

How does the baby produce these steroids? The developing baby's adrenal glands are larger than its kidneys. Even after birth they are still relatively large – about twenty times their relative size in an adult – and so have to undergo a period of downsizing until they are the 'right' size. One of their chief functions during fetal life, however, is to semi-assemble steroid hormones before passing them over to the placenta where the manufacturing into fully fledged oestrogens takes place. Roughly ten times more steroids go from baby to mother than the other way round. Passing incomplete steroids over to the mother is cunning because it means that the baby is protected from the harmful effects of the steroids.

Another ingenious arrangement is in the way that the baby is protected from the mother's stress responses. Pregnant women seem serene and untroubled. This is not just the effect of the barbiturate-like progesterone, it's also because their hormonal response to stress is dramatically damped down, mainly by the action of oxytocin in the brain. The release of corticotrophins (the hormones that tell the mother's adrenals to produce stress hormones) is dramatically reduced, especially in the last trimester of pregnancy. Things that should send stress hormones soaring in non-pregnant women don't.

On the other hand, if the mother *is* stressed in pregnancy, it seems to reset the baby's stress response for the rest of its life, and it develops hyperarousal – an abnormally high cortisol response to normal stressors. Continued high levels of cortisol are associated with a variety of adult disorders, including cardiovascular disease and also depression. This fits closely with the Barker hypothesis, developed by David Barker and his colleagues at Southampton

University, which says that adult health is programmed by conditions in the womb. The more a baby is stressed (this also includes things like poor nutrition, poor blood flow) during pregnancy, the more likely he or she is to develop problems such as cardiovascular disease or diabetes in later life. Damping down the mother's stress response means that programming isn't triggered unless it's really necessary.

If this is true, and if nature does indeed so assiduously protect babies from the mother's stress hormones, prescribing additional corticosteroids during pregnancy could disturb the baby's hypothalamus sufficiently to reset its programming, perhaps causing poor health in later life. Of course women are not usually given large doses of these type of drugs during pregnancy except in one situation. If it becomes apparent that a woman is going to go into premature labour, or if the baby has to be delivered early, the mother is given large doses of corticosteroids to help mature the baby's lungs and prevent it from suffering life-threatening breathing problems. Doctors are now beginning to wonder whether this treatment might be at the expense of the baby's future health. For this reason, there is now more caution about using these drugs unless absolutely necessary (though they can be life-savers) and the health of children who have been treated is being monitored on a long-term basis.

Of course hormones are involved in the growth of the baby too. You might assume that growth hormone would be essential but deficiencies of it during pregnancy are not associated with anything more than minimal reductions in fetal weight or length. Deficiency or excess of insulin, however, is a totally different matter. Diabetic women whose insulin is poorly controlled in pregnancy can have very large babies – 4.5 kg (nearly 10lb) and more, compared to the British average of 3.3 kg (7lb 2oz). This is called macrosomia. Too little insulin, on the other hand, and the babies do not grow properly. Leprechaunism is a type of dwarfism in which the baby, as the name implies, is very tiny, has elfin features and large low-set ears. It's caused by a genetic defect of insulin receptors.

We've seen how hormone levels at conception may influence sex selection. Hormone levels during pregnancy also have a profound effect on gender, altering appearance to female (despite the chromosomes saying male) and affecting brain type.

Gender Development

You don't have to believe that men come from Mars and women from Venus to appreciate that there's a difference between the way that men and women think and act. It's obvious right from the very start, as any parent knows. Boys and girls are simply different. It's not simply gender stereotyping to say that boys are more interested in construction toys, cars and rough play as toddlers. Little girls *do* prefer to play caring, sharing games with dolls and teddies. On the whole they don't like the rough and tumble that so engages little boys. These differences become, if anything, more marked with age.

Women are much better at judging social situations and are more sensitive to facial expressions than men. They worry about how other people are feeling, putting themselves in their shoes (empathizing) and are keen to chat and share intimacy. Men are better at working out how things work (systemizing), be it washing machines, computer programs or armies; they prefer games and gadgets. They may start collecting things – football stats, CDs, beer mats – a hobby which is often a complete mystery to women. At the same time the appeal of watching soaps on TV and the concept of shopping for pleasure is mystifying men. Most men will run a mile before they do the 'talking about problems' thing.

You can look at gender in several different ways. Being XX or XY makes you female or male, of course, but there's actually more to it than that. For instance, you could be genetically female, genitally female (i.e. you have a normal vagina), but if the hormones produced by your sex organs (gonads) have been more male than usual, these would influence your brain type and thus your sex-typical behaviour.

Or you could be a man, chromosomally and genitally male, who develops female-typical behaviour (and appearance) because of more female hormones in the womb. The mechanism that turns the embryo's genetic sex into the adult male or female depends on an immensely complex interplay of genetic, psychological, social and, naturally, hormonal factors. The chief hormonal factor is the influence of testosterone in the womb.

There are supposed to be five characteristics of the male brain type: aggression, competition, self-assertion, self-confidence and self-reliance. All these are highly correlated with adult testosterone level, whether in men or women. The characteristics of the female brain type are better skills at language, sensory awareness, memory, social awareness and relationships. Male and female brain types are organized in a different way too. For instance, visual spatial perception is found in the right hemispheres in men but in the right *and* left hemisphere in women. Women use both hemispheres for vocabulary, men use only their left. This is dramatically demonstrated by the after-effects of stroke. Women who have sustained damage to their left hemisphere are less likely to have language problems (disphasia) than men. Even if they do have some degree of disphasia, they tend to recover language more quickly than men, perhaps because the other hemisphere is taking over some of the functions of the damaged part. In people who have brain damage following accidents, left hemisphere damage is more likely to cause language problems in men, whereas in women, language test scores tend not to be affected by whether the damage is to the left or right.

This is not only about gender. Some men are empathizers – about one in five – and about one in ten women are systemizers. Nor is this about homosexuality – you don't have to be a gay man to know the lyrics to Judy Garland songs and be able to match upholstery fabrics. This is about brain type. Logically, there should be an extreme female brain type, driven by an excess of oestrogen in the womb. Baron Cohen speculates that such a woman might be an endlessly patient psychotherapist, or alternatively a woman who is completely at sea with anything mechanical and just stands there looking helpless while men fall about wanting to help her.

There are three periods during development when there is a surge of testosterone. In the next chapter, I'll be exploring the second period, during adolescence. Now let's examine what occurs between the eighth and twenty-fourth week of pregnancy and how it influences gender.

The default gender in the womb is female, which is perhaps hardly surprising given that the womb is an environment awash with female hormones. A genetically male fetus will therefore develop the female form of sexual organs until 'maleness' is switched on by the SRY gene on the Y chromosome, and the fetal testis starts to develop and then produce testosterone. Incidentally a functioning ovary is not needed to appear to be female, whereas a functioning testis is essential for a man.

A clue about the effect of hormones in the womb comes from the Diethylstilboestrol (DES) tragedy. DES is a synthetic oestrogen. From the end of the Second World War on, it was prescribed to pregnant women mainly in the US, in the mistaken belief that it would prevent miscarriage. At the time it was thought that miscarriages were caused by a drop in oestrogen, although such a drop is now known to be a result of miscarriage, not the cause of it. In fact, DES was a potent carcinogen and twenty years on was discovered to cause a rare and sometimes fatal type of vaginal cancer in some young women who had been exposed to it in the womb, as well as infertility in others. It was withdrawn from use in 1971. The cancers affected females but there was also a curious effect on males exposed to DES: they were more likely to show female-typical behaviour such as enacting social themes in their play or caring for dolls.

There are also natural variations in hormone levels which provide clues to the effects in the womb. Boys with a condition called idiopathic hypogonadotrophic hypogonadism (IHH), in which the testes are very small, are poor at systemizing. Babies born with congenital adrenal hyperplasia (CAH), a disease that sends their adrenals into hyperdrive, over-produce a type of testosterone. Affected girls have stronger systemizing abilities. Curiously, affected boys are not simply better than other boys at systemizing because of those extra androgens – the rule seems to be that very high or very low androgen levels are bad news and that in the middle is best.

Professor Simon Baron Cohen, a psychologist and Director of the Autism Research Centre at Cambridge University, has a special interest in male/female brain types, particularly in relation to autism, and wanted to find out whether levels of testosterone in the womb affected behaviour. Luckily, the University hospital is a regional centre for amniocentesis (a procedure in which fluid is taken from the amniotic sac for analysis) and once the necessary tests had been done, it was their policy to freeze the remainder of the sample. Baron Cohen and his team contacted women whose samples were still in the deep freeze, who now had toddlers and were happy to bring them in for an assessment of their behaviour. The researchers found that the higher the levels of pre-natal testosterone in the amniotic fluid, the less eye contact the toddlers made, and the smaller their vocabulary. These toddlers were seen again when they were four years old. By this time, those children that had had the highest level of pre-natal testoerone had lower social skills and more restricted interests than those who had had lower levels of testosterone in their bath of amniotic fluid.

Fetal testosterone clearly affects the brain in some way and therefore influences behaviour for the rest of the baby's life. In a nutshell, the more you have in the womb, the more of a systemizer you are; the less you have, the more of an empathizer you are. While of course baby boys produce more testosterone, baby girls also produce it, some almost to the levels of the least producing boys. Both sexes are subjected to the hormonal environment in the mother, which is yet another source of testosterone (and indeed oestrogen). In addition to the mother's natural levels of testosterone (which vary from woman to woman), more may come from other sources.

For instance, vigorous exercise during pregnancy raises testosterone levels, although sustained exercise, such as a long run, lowers testosterone. If a woman is under a great deal of stress during pregnancy, as a result, for example, of bereavement or war, testosterone levels are increased.

Norman Geschwind, a legendary US neurologist and teacher, believed that fetal testosterone has an effect on the rate of growth of the two hemispheres of the brain. The right hemisphere is involved in spatial ability, the left in communication. If the right side of the brain develops faster, systemizing and spatial skills will be favoured; if it's the left side, it will improve the ability to empathize and communicate. One of the effects of a right-side surge, caused by testosterone, is that men are less attuned to words spoken in their left ear than those in their right. This is called the right ear advantage because auditory connections are greatest on the contralateral side of the brain. You might want to rearrange your pillow-talking positions ... Part of the evidence for differential hemisphere growth comes from the Wada test, in which the hemispheres of the brain can be put to sleep individually with an anaesthetic. Women's fluency with words is reduced no matter which side is 'dark'. Men's verbals only decrease if the left hemisphere is asleep.

Another interesting twist are the findings of Doreen Kimura, a neuropsychologist at the University of Western Ontario, who identified a relationship beween gender-related behaviour and body asymmetry. Men and women with bigger right testicles or breasts tend to exhibit more masculine traits, while those with left-sided dominance show more feminine characteristics. Norman Geschwind also hypothesized that fetal androgens promote growth not just of the right hemisphere, but also of the right side of the body. Indeed, some, but not all, studies find that in men the right foot is larger than the left, and the right testicle is larger than the left one, whereas in women the left foot and left ovary are larger than the right ones.

You don't have to strip off to notice these asymmetries. Your fingers display them, as does your face. More angular faces are produced by higher levels of fetal testosterone, which promotes the lateral growth of cheekbones and chin (the chiselled masculine jaw which was mentioned earlier). A rounder face, with more prominent lips and higher eyebrows, speaks of lesser levels of testosterone. Facial features are a nightmare to measure in a consistent reproducible way but John Manning, an evolutionary biologist who worked mainly at the University of Manchester, has shown that prenatal testosterone stimulates growth of the fourth finger (look at your left hand, palm up, with your thumb as No. 1 finger, your fourth is your ring finger). Oestrogen promotes the growth of the second finger (the index finger). A low 2D:4D ratio (fourth finger longer than the second) is a marker for high womb testosterone. A high 2D:4D ratio (second finger longer than the fourth), may be a marker for a womb environment low in testosterone.

This is fascinating stuff and finger lengths have been used to predict all sorts of things, for instance, greater proclivity towards homosexuality and higher music aptitude (in those with high 2D:4D ratios) as well as differences in fertility, although this seems to stretch the science to its limit (if not well beyond it). There is a very substantial overlap between the sexes with respect to digit ratio, far more so than there is with height, and the ratio varies with geography and race, so one suspects there is more than just fetal testosterone at work here. Nevertheless, digit ratio is clear in, say, girls with congenital adrenal hyperplasia (CAH) – that's where the girl is exposed to high levels of androgen in the womb and also in those with Asperger's syndrome (AS), a type of autism. It is to autism, and Simon Baron Cohen, that we now return.

Autism

We have seen that there is a male brain type and that this brain type is not about gender; rather, it is about the level of testosterone during fetal life. Baron Cohen, whose work on autism is highly respected, believes that one form of autism, Asperger's syndrome, represents an extreme of the male brain type.

Asperger's syndrome is often called high-functioning autism, because intelligence is not affected – in fact, it may be higher than normal. Indeed, some AS individuals may be supremely gifted, but they also have great difficulties with relationships and with empathy. Most of us can 'read' situations to varying degrees. We have an understanding of what or how someone else may be thinking and we are then able to adjust what we say or do accordingly, but those with Asperger's have great difficulty in 'reading' other people. They are, in Baron Cohen's words, 'mind blind'. They also have a tendency to blurt out the truth – 'you have a nasty big nose' – because they cannot understand, as we do, that there are some things that you shouldn't say. They are most comfortable when they are in control of their world and will seek to master every last detail of a 'system' because this provides predictability. There are rules and laws which govern how a system behaves, unlike people whose behaviour is totally mystifying. In those professions where attention to detail is everything, people with Asperger's can thrive. They flourish in professions like physics, engineering and maths, where their social skills are less important. Isaac Newton, Nobel prize-winning physicist Paul Dirac and Albert Einstein are all examples of supremely successful scientists who probably all had Asperger's syndrome.

What's interesting about AS is that there are ten males to every female with the condition. In tests of systemizing, men score better than women and those with autism score highest of all. On empathizing, women generally score better than men, while those with autism score worst of all. Of course, levels of testosterone in the womb do not explain all forms of autism, which is a neuro-developmental disorder with a strong genetic component.

Eye contact is another thing that children with autism find dif-ficult. As we will see later, oxytocin is released when a mother looks at her baby and helps with bonding and developing maternal behav-iour. It has been suggested recently that excess oxytocin (derived from synthetic oxytocin used during delivery to hasten labour) may somehow affect the baby's normal oxytocin receptors, downregu-lating them and so contributing to the development of autism spectrum disorders. Certainly, oxytocin is crucial in social behaviour and attachment. Mice specially bred to have no oxytocin, despite normal development, seem to have trouble recognizing their family members, even though they have normal eyesight and smell. Nevertheless, the theory that synthetic oxytocin actually causes autism seems highly unlikely.

Birth

You'd think that we would know exactly how labour starts by now. Researchers certainly know pretty much all there is to know about what triggers labour in sheep, but in humans it's still a bit of a mystery, despite years of intense study. Being born too soon is a major cause of 70 per cent of baby deaths and 50 per cent of cerebral palsy in babies, and better knowledge of the mechanics of normal labour would also lead to an understanding of how to intervene to prevent premature labour.

It was always presumed that it must be the mother's hormones that mattered. Today it's thought that those of the baby are more important. The child dictates, not the mother. For anyone pregnant as they read this, the bad news is that this is a pattern set for the next two decades of your life.

The hormone that was initially identified as the birth initiator was oxytocin, which is produced by both the mother's and the baby's pituitary glands around the time of birth. This is one of those unusual hormones that comes from the back or posterior pituitary, rather than the front of this gland, and is of the protein and peptide family. Oxytocin is the hormone of attraction as we've seen, but it is also the hormone of birth and what's called the milk let-down reflex. It is so powerful that a mother merely has to see her baby, or hear the sound of it crying, to prompt the release of oxytocin, which then squeezes the breast tissue and forces milk from her nipples. We'll see later how oxytocin also affects the mother's psychological state too.

For many years it was thought that rising levels of oxytocin, produced by the mother from her pituitary, were the trigger for labour, or, alternatively, that the womb became more and more sensitive to oxytocin as pregnancy advanced. It wasn't until the 1960s and the development of better test methods, that it was discovered that there was no sudden increase in oxytocin prior to birth. However, there is a flood of it late on in labour, stimulated by the stretching of the birth canal by the baby's head. Remember that when the placenta is delivered, there is effectively a big open wound inside the womb where the placenta has been ripped from its wall. When you cut yourself, applying pressure will help stop the bleeding; if the womb does not contract down hard after delivery of the placenta, there is a risk of a life-threatening haemorrhage. A surge of oxytocin at this stage ensures that the womb squeezes down tight.

If you are waiting for your baby to be born, those last weeks can be interminable. Every day past the due date is agonizing. There are many old wives' tales about how to bring on labour. One of the oldest is that of twiddling the nipples, or even brushing them. One elderly GP I knew told his expectant mums to use a nail brush on their nipples to promote the release of oxytocin, which is certainly produced by suckling. In truth, nipple-twiddling probably doesn't actually do that much in terms of speeding the onset of labour – but it's fun and at least it gives you something to do of a winter's evening.

Passionate sex – which is tricky at term when you look and feel like a beached whale – is probably more effective. Semen contains prostaglandins, or 'pre-hormones' and these help to 'ripen' the cervix. Perhaps more importantly, the rhythmic contractions of orgasm, initiated by oxytocin, may set up contractions which refuse then to settle and disappear, and which, by positive feedback, may get labour established.

Another hormone that may play a part is progesterone, whose levels drop as birth approaches. Certainly progesterone inhibits prolactin during prenancy, which ensures milk production after birth. It is more likely, however, that the drop in progesterone is to do with releasing control of prolactin rather than itself initiating labour.

So what is the baby's role in organizing its exit from the womb? Could its master gland, the pituitary, be directing operations, rather than the mother's? Certainly fetal oxytocin is produced in great quantity, but, just as in the mother, it occurs around the time of delivery, not before. There could be a role for another of the fetal pituitary hormones, ACTH, from the anterior pituitary. ACTH acts to gear up production of the stress hormone cortisol. Animal studies in sheep have shown that without a fetal pituitary gland there is no natural onset of labour. If ACTH is injected, lots of cortisol is made by the fetal adrenal gland and labour starts prematurely.

In humans, there is an abnormality called anencephaly in which much of the brain is missing, including the pituitary. It's in the same family of problems as spina bifida and is incompatible with life. It's usually detected very early in pregnancy, using ultrasound. Some women choose to terminate the pregnancy, some continue with it. Is it possible that, as with sheep, pregnancy is prolonged in these human pregnancies too?

Some people, such as Roger Smith of the University of Newcastle in Australia, believe that labour is genetically pre-programmed, pointing out that the tendency to have premature births can run in families. He believes that it is the placenta that acts as a countdown clock and that the cascade of events begins with placental release of corticotrophin releasing hormone (CRH). Every woman has her own unique profile of CRH production during pregnancy, which might suggest a personal pregnancy timetable. What CRH does is enhance the production of 'negative' receptors that block progesterones's actions. Whilst at the same time promoting the effect of oestrogen by upping the production of its receptors. Remember that receptors are Harry Potterish, appearing and disappearing. It is believed that the negative progesterone receptors, which inhibit its actions suddenly start to appear close to labour, and once the effects of progesterone begin to fall, the womb just gets more and more twitchy, its musculature less and less able to stop itself contracting, until labour begins. One suspects that there isn't just one switch for labour, but a cascade of them.

Dads-to-be sometimes have symptoms of pregnancy such as nausea, weight gain and mood swings. This is called couvade, or sympathetic pregnancy. Prolactin is highest in men in the week before the birth and testosterone production falls after birth. Paternal prolactin is positively associated with those men who report couvade symptoms. It seems that the same hormones involved in bonding in the mother are also changing in the expectant father, probably to ensure that he helps care for his child. Researchers were surprised to discover this effect in male tamarin monkeys. Their prolactin started to increase some two weeks before their young were born. The level of prolactin seemed to have little to do with how much time the monkeys spent with their offspring, and researchers speculated that prolactin may help fathers tolerate the presence of infants, thus keeping them from being harmed by the father.

In a baby boy, there is a surge of testosterone to almost adult levels within hours of birth. By the end of the first week, this outpouring ceases, only for there to be a further whoosh a month later. In the first weeks of life, a baby boy has as much plasma testosterone as a healthy red-blooded twenty-five year old. But by the time he is six months old the system has damped down, remaining quiet until puberty. Meanwhile, in baby girls, follicle stimulating hormone (FSH) rises after the first week of life to levels equivalent to that of a menopausal woman, and then declines over the next three years, before rising again at puberty. We don't really have an explanation for these surges and falls of hormones in babies.

The placenta pumps out industrial quantities of hormones during pregnancy. One job they have to do is to squash ovulation completely. They're pretty successful. The levels of follicle stimulating hormone (that's the one that sets the follicles off in the race to release an egg each month) and luteinising hormone (the one that triggers ovulation) are suppressed to less than 1 per cent of normal levels. Once the placenta has been delivered, there is a catastrophic drop in hormone levels – which has many consequences.

Some 70 per cent of mothers will experience the blues during the first ten days after delivery. Many women do become quite irrational. Someone will kindly offer a cup of tea and you burst into tears; you abuse your spouse, quarrel with the mother-in-law (although perhaps that's nothing to do with hormones) and may find yourself alternately weepy and euphoric. It has been suggested that this is all about hormones, particuarly the catastrophic drop in progesterone. While it is true that those most likely to be severely affected will have suffered the steepest drop in progesterone, pre- and post-birth, remain to be convinced that the baby blues is simply about hormones. Try keeping a man awake for twenty-four hours while subjecting him to intense pain from a life-changing event. Then see what his mood is like while he is deprived of sleep, made to leak from every orifice, while imposing on him all the relatives you've ever known who arrive at your home expecting you to be nice to them.

For most women, however, the blues usually pass quickly. Of more concern are those 10 per cent of women who develop more long-lasting post-natal depression. Here, although everyone has tried very hard to find a biological basis, hormones stubbornly refuse to be implicated, with no obvious differences in levels between affected and non-affected women. Most of the risk factors seem to be psychosocial, with previous depression and obstetric complication important, and social adversity factors, particularly lack of support, paramount. Giving women progesterone might seem logical, given the way that it falls, but the evidence does not support its use and in fact synthetic progestogens may make things worse. Some people believe that natural progesterone has better results, but this is by no means proven. There is some evidence that for a small group of women oestrogens may be helpful. Nevertheless cognitive behavioural therapy and other psychological interventions are of more benefit.

Hormone levels actually return to normal remarkably quickly. The downside is that this means you can get pregnant again remarkably quickly too. I once sat next to a man at a dinner and remarked on how close his children were in age. He confided: 'If you have a private room, you might as well use it for something useful.' Part of me wanted to slap the toad, and I do remember saying rather too crisply that it wasn't physiologically possible. Actually his tale might not have been as apocryphal as it sounds (although in my view it says more about his wife being remarkable than him). To get pregnant, you have to ovulate, of course, and normally speaking you've got no FSH worth speaking of with which to conjure up a follicle in the week after delivery. By four weeks after delivery, your FSH is right back up there again and in charge of its unruly mob once more. The other hormone you need for ovulation is LH, which is slower in recovery. What's interesting is work that suggests that the more you sleep, the more quickly LH gets back to its normal duties.

Within three months, 70 per cent of non-breastfeeding women have had a return of their periods. But it is possible to have immediate resumption of ovarian activity. I realize that what follows is on a par with those dire warnings in sex lessons at school where, with a voice of doom, a teacher told you that it was possible to get pregnant if a sperm came within spitting distance of you, at any time of your cycle – a case of the technically possible, vanishingly rare scenario being used to frighten you into avoiding sperm, spitting or otherwise, for all time. However a Dutch case study did record the plight of a twenty year old in whom a 13.5-week fetus was demonstrated by ultrasound just 15.5 weeks after delivery. I should make the point here that pregnancy dating always includes two weeks in which you weren't pregnant (because it is dated back to your last period – or birth in this case – even though technically you didn't get pregnant till you ovulated two weeks or so later). To put this into perspective, it would mean that your children would be in the same class at school and that you could be going into labour at a time when your first baby isn't even sitting up properly yet. At least with twins, it's only one delivery.

What about the effect of breastfeeding on hormones? Breast-feeding definitely delays the return of periods, although this is hugely variable. What counts is the duration of feeding and to a lesser extent, night suckling and your nutritional status. For western women, duration refers to the length of each feed as well the months for which breastfeeding is continued. The hormone at work here is prolactin.

Prolactin is another of those hormones that comes from the anterior rather than posterior pituitary. It's an extraordinary hormone. For a start it is an almost dead ringer for growth hormone. In fact, it was not until 1971 than people knew definitively that prolactin and growth hormone (which also has an effect on milk production) were two distinct hormones in humans, not one. Prolactin is an ancient molecule whose original function was to maintain salt and water balance in fish, although it can be traced further back, being associated in snails with sexual behaviour. Prolactin also occurs in pigeons.

You might wonder what a hormone that stimulates lactation in humans is doing in birds who don't have breasts (or at least not of the lactating kind). In birds, prolactin works with oestrogen to produce those odd bald brood patches whose appearance coincides with the arrival of eggs in the nest. In doves and pigeons, prolactin stimulates the production of the curiously named crop milk. Actually it's not milk at all – just a whitish looking sludge of cells from the inside of part of the stomach (the crop sac), which is regurgitated and fed, by both parents, to the fledgling squabs.

Just as in humans, prolactin in birds has a dampening effect on reproduction. Cooing is what counts for foreplay amonge male doves – and it's driven by the male's hormones. Castrate a male dove and it will no longer coo. Give it a shot of prolactin, and the same thing happens. A silent dove. High levels of prolactin may also be one reason why breastfeeding women feel less sexual desire in the early months after delivery, although sore bits and exhaustion probably play a larger part.

Today, tests to measure the level of prolactin in the blood are carried out using radioimmunoassays (RIA), which use the competition between radioactively labelled and non-radioactively labelled substances to determine the concentration of the unlabelled one. But this sort of testing didn't arrive on the scene until the early 1970s. A mere thirty years ago, in vivo bioassays (a bioassay is a test that uses another animal) for prolactin involved injecting a human sample into a pigeon and measuring the weight of its crop sac to see if it had increased – a procedure which seems almost medieval to us now.

That lactation in women is under hormonal control was convincingly demonstrated by the case of a pair of Siamese twins, Rosalie and Josefa Blazek. The twins were joined in the sacral region and shared the lower 3 cm of the urethra, the vagina and the lower 5 cm of the rectum. Rosalie became pregnant, and while only she had most of the symptoms of pregnancy, breast development occurred in them both. After delivery of a healthy boy weighing 3 kg in April 1910, both secreted milk – although both refused to breastfeed.

Prolactin maintains milk production, although it is oxytocin that is responsible for letting the milk out through the nipple. It is the act of suckling that both releases oxytocin to obtain the baby's present meal and orders up future meals by stimulating the release of prolactin. Oxytocin also acts within the brain to increase bonding. The 'look of love' between mother and feeding baby is almost certainly prompted and enhanced by oxytocin. You'd think that it would be the fall-off in prolactin levels when the baby is no longer suckling as much that presages the return to normal ovulation. Curiously, it's not the amount of prolactin that seems to be important, it's how it is secreted that counts. It is released in pulsed doses but the pulsing gets way out of kilter during breastfeeding. Only when suckling is reduced and the pulses get back to their normal rhythm does ovulation return.

Prolactin, originally thought to be simply a milk hormone in humans, seems to have far more widespread actions than originally thought. Once again we return to sex. One of the side effects of some medications taken by those with schizophrenia is a big hike in circulating prolactin. In women, as you might expect, it causes milk secretion, breast engorgement and menstrual disturbances. Men develop breast tissue but also have reduced sperm production because prolactin forces down levels of oestrogen and testosterone. Both men and women have sexual dysfunction and in the long term are at risk of decreased bone density and, it is thought, cardio-vascular disease. Significantly for these people, who are already facing one major mental health condition, elevated prolactin is also associated with depression. So here you have an example of the enormously broad sweep of hormones. First, they interact – one affecting levels of another, or others – and second, their effects are not just on their supposed primary tissue but all over the place, including the brain where they affect mood and behaviour. In the next chapter, we'll see what happens to behaviour during the hormonal mania that is adolescence.

CHAPTER THREE

HORMONE EXPLOSIONS 2
The Teenage Years

Something very strange happens at puberty, when truckloads of hormones begin arriving by the day. Children who were sweet, helpful and good fun to be around, turn almost overnight into grunting creatures who wear nothing but black, lie in bed till noon and consume 5,000-calorie snacks (and still say they're hungry). They preface every request for help, or an invitation to go somewhere with their parents and siblings, by 'Do I have to?'; become the most completely self-centred, self-obsessed and selfish creatures on the planet – until they go to other people's homes, in which case they are perfectly adorable. They are spotty, start – and I mean this kindly – to smell and grow out of everything they have in the space of a few months. Their boredom threshold plummets and they do not seem able to concentrate on anything for more than five minutes at a time. You begin to wonder whether your child is a changeling, swapped with your own by an alien from the Planet MTV while you weren't looking.

Teenagers are trapped in limbo – neither children nor adults: an excruciating mix of vulnerability and potential, which by turns engages, inspires and alienates adults, where everything they do has a high-intensity feel about it. We know this because our own adolescent experience – our first kiss, the first time we fell in love, the rush of first-time driving – still burns brightly thirty or forty years on.

However there is a darker side too: soaring rates of serious accidents, illicit use of drugs or alcohol, risky sexual behaviour and its consequences, and the first signs of emotional disorders which may be lifelong. Teenagers seem to be the very embodiment of hormonal mayhem – or are they? This chapter investigates the truth about teenagers and hormones – and it's not what you expect.

All Growed Up

Puberty is an extraordinary event and human beings are lucky in that they only have to go through it once, which is not the norm in the rest of the animal kingdom. Most animals do not become sexually active and then remain so, as we do, but confine their sexual activity to a single breeding season. This means pretty much starting from scratch every year – new plumage or antlers, a huge increase in testicle size, commencement of courtship behaviour, territory marking, even an increase in song repertoire if you are a songbird. All these events are orchestrated by hormones and preceded by a hormone rush, just like the one experienced by teenagers. If you look in your garden in the spring and see blue tits scrapping among themselves while singing their heads off, they're hormonal.

Another aspect of human puberty is that all other animals, including great apes, go straight from juvenile to adult. In humans, however, there is a stage between the appearance of reproductive hormones and the prime reproductive age. Boys become fertile at around thirteen, while they are still puny and unappealing. Girls acquire a womanly shape at puberty, yet are relatively infertile for several years thereafter. The conjunction of top male specimen at around twenty and fully reproductive female at eighteen is reflected in the average age of first birth across all cultures of nineteen years of age.

Let's look first at the hormonal changes that lead a child through and beyond puberty, into independence, physical maturity and the ability to reproduce. These stages unfold in an orderly and highly integrated way, and while the whole process can be delayed or advanced, it will still follow that same prescribed pattern. If there is puberty without growth, or the other way around, there is almost certainly something amiss in the hormone department.

There are three main hormonal elements to puberty. Alterations in the secretions of the adrenal gland, differences in secretions of the ovaries or testes and changes relating to growth hormone. These are all interlinked – for instance, increasing production of testosterone and oestrogen primes the pituitary gland to produce an increase in growth hormone.

The first hormone event which will lead to puberty is largely hidden from us. Between the ages of six and eight, the adrenal gland starts to step up secretion of androgens such as DHEA (dehydro-epiandrosterone), which the body uses as construction material for the manufacture of other steroids. These androgens will stimulate the growth of sebaceous glands, which produce the skin-lubricating fluid sebum. This results in greasier skin and body odour and also primes hair follicles in those areas where pubic hair will later begin to grow. This is called adrenarche. Parents first notice this at their kids' parties, when twenty sweaty seven year olds rampaging in a confined space (your sitting room) are noticeably whiffy in a way that they were not when younger. The increase in adrenal hormone levels continues steadily until they peak in the mid-twenties.

In adult men, and in women of reproductive age, the hypo-thalamus is constantly secreting pulsed doses of gonadotrophin releasing hormone (GnRH), which tells the pituitary to secrete hormones, which then act on ovary and testicle to produce the reproductive hormones which will ensure a supply of sperm and eggs. These hormones as we have seen also influence our behaviour profoundly, making us sexual beings. But in childhood, the hypo-thalamus does not secrete GnRH, and as a result there are not only minimal levels of reproductive hormones in children but little or no sexual behaviour either. It is as if there were a brake on the hypo-thalamus. True puberty starts when the brakes are taken off and the hypothalamus is permitted to begin the pulsed secretion of gonado-trophin releasing hormone. The pattern of this hormone secretion is more important than the total amount of hormone secreted. If, as in some medical conditions, GnRH is 'on' all the time, rather than being delivered in pulsed doses every ninety minutes or so, surprisingly, puberty will be delayed. GnRH tells the anterior pituitary to produce both follicle stimulating hormone (FSH) and luteinising hormone (LH). You may be more familiar with these hormones as the ones controlling your monthly cycles, but FSH and LH in men control production of sperm and male hormones. This is an illustration of the way in which a hormone can have radically different effects depending on the target organ or tissue.

In boys, LH secretion stimulates the production of testosterone by cells in the testes. LH too is secreted in pulsed doses. At first, there is a very clear daily pattern, with peak production occurring during sleep, especially between midnight and 8 a.m. As puberty progresses, LH is also secreted during the day. The production of testosterone mirrors that of LH, being at first, greatest at night. Simultaneously, levels of the substances that keep testosterone under lock and key in the bloodstream – sex hormone binding globulins – decrease, thus making even more testosterone available, fifty times more than was experienced before puberty. That's some hormone rush. The earliest visible sign of sexual development in boys is enlargement of the testicles. The penis also begins to lengthen in early puberty, and later thickens.

In girls, the first sign of changes in gonadotrophin secretion are seen in levels of FSH, rather than luteinising hormone (which is the one that prompts ovulation). The effect of FSH is to stimulate the growth of follicles in the ovary which begin to produce oestrogen. It also ups the activity of an enzyme, aromatase, which converts androgens to oestrogens. Before puberty, pulses of LH occur at night. These are irregular, but as time passes they become progressively larger and more regular. Just as with boys, LH is then secreted during the day too. The secretion of LH at night is not linked to darkness but to dreaming (REM) sleep. This can be demonstrated very easily. If you blindfold a teenager during the day, so that they experience darkness but are not asleep, there is no alteration in the amount of LH secreted. If, however, sleeping periods are switched, so that normal sleep takes place during the day and activity occurs throughout the night, LH secretion will then also take place during the day, coinciding with dreaming sleep. Oestrogens are also pulsed. Peak secretion of oestrogens in teenage girls is between 6 and 10 in the morning. These rhythms of secretion disappear once ovulation is established.

The time between onset of these GnRH pulses and the first period in girls is relatively short. But having a period for the first time does not mean that the girl is fertile. Regular cycling may take three years to establish and although sporadic periods occur they are frequently associated with anovular cycles (in which no egg is released). This may be the source of that well-known old wives' tale about not getting pregnant the first time you do it. If there are teenagers reading this book, your mantra should be you can get pregnant at any time of your cycle, in any position. I have never understood why it is that the tune should suddenly change at thirty-five when you are told that you can only get pregnant during your fertile period. More likely to – yes, but definitely not 'only'. Be warned.

Once oestrogens and testosterone begin to be produced, it is their impact on body form which provides the most dramatic expression of adolescence. Oestrogen stimulates growth of the womb and breast but also determines the shape of the female figure by some judicious rearranging of the deposition of fat. In boys, the consequence of testosterone is also to sculpt the body, increasing lean body mass and shaping features as well as promoting body hair and beard growth. Oestrogen and testosterone also promote fusion at the end of the long bones, which will eventually signal the termination of their period of rapid growth.

Spots

Acne is common in both sexes during adolescence. Mothers tell their teenagers that their spots are the result of eating too much chocolate or fatty food. Not enough fresh air (as in, you've been in your room too long) is also proffered as a cause. Actually it's the fault of your hormones, not your diet. There is an abnormal response in the skin to normal levels of testosterone in the blood. This has a profound effect on appearance for some unlucky people. The response is self-limiting and goes away with time, but there is no way of predicting how long it will take – it can be a couple of years or decades. It may leave deep, pitted scarring. Adolescents, although the most likely sufferers, aren't the only ones to get acne. It is often reported, for the first time, by women in their thirties. Typically, they also report a highly stressed lifestyle. In this case, stress causes an increase in the level of male hormones, bringing back teenage spots.

Growth

In the last chapter we established that the growth of babies in the womb is not wholly dependent on growth hormone and that nutrition is an important factor. However, increasingly growth hormone – as you would expect from its name – does dictate and coordinate growth in the baby, promoting increases in bone, soft tissue and organ size. A tiny baby has no growth hormone receptors in its tissues, but these begin to appear when it is about seven months of age and it is at this age that GH begins its effect.

Height is one of the most heritable body factors and if you come from a tall family, the odds are that you too will be tall. Smaller parents are likely to have less tall children – still perfectly proportioned, just built on a smaller scale. Your eventual height is influenced by many different things: whether or not your mother smoked during pregnancy, her nutrition in pregnancy, whether you got enough to eat as a child, whether you were seriously ill or emotionally deprived, stressed or abused, what illnesses you had, to name but a few.

Season also affects growth – which is mediated through the hormone of sleep, melatonin – both in children and in babies before birth. A large study of over a million Danish babies showed that those babies born in April were on average 2.2 mm taller than those born in December. This confirms earlier work from Austria showing a height variation of up to 6 mm depending on month of birth, with once again the tallest children being born in the spring.

Crucially, the mother manages to switch off some of the paternal genes involved in growth during pregnancy – which means that a 5' woman can have a 6' 6" man's baby without the baby's feet bursting out of the womb. It's the same mechanism that allows Great Danes to impregnate spaniels, but the mother spaniel not to expire in the process.

Adolescence is marked by a huge surge in growth hormone production. It starts soon after the initiation of gonadotrophin releasing hormone secretion. The relationship between these two hormones is an indirect one, however, involving oestrogen. The idea that a female hormone is driving growth in boys as well as girls is counterintuitive at first, but it explains much about the gender differences in growth and why girls grow earlier and faster than boys: it's because they have oestrogens which pump up production of growth hormone. In boys, the enzyme aromatase converts testosterone to oestrogen. That this is key to growth is shown by those rare cases in which children have gene mutations affecting either aromatase or oestrogen receptors, whose growth patterns are radically altered.

The secretion of growth hormone is carefully timetabled in a pattern that persists through puberty. Growth hormone is released principally at night during sleep, in short bursts every one to two hours during the deep sleep phase. So when your mum says, if you don't go to bed now you won't grow up to be big and strong, she's right. If the onset of sleep is delayed, so is the onset of growth hormone release. Children who are deprived of sleep are smaller than they should be.

It is apparent to all that there are big gender differences in growth hormone during puberty. These accounted for my own misery at school. I was 5′ 10″ at twelve, which was to be my final height. Forced to do ballroom dancing lessons with boys of the same age from a nearby boys' school, I found myself towering over them by what appeared to be several feet. As we whirled about, they missed the overhead beams in the centuries-old building in Winchester which passed for a dance hall, whereas I did not. After two hideously embarrassing lessons, I was excused all further dancing duties. One of my former dancing partners is now six inches taller than me (and still as poor on the dancefloor as he was then). Thank God my mother smoked forty cigarettes a day during pregnancy, or else I would have been 6′ 3″.

Before the onset of the teenage growth spurt, boys grow very slightly faster than girls, but girls' growth spurt starts about two years before that of boys between twelve and fourteen. For some four years, girls are on average taller than boys. But by adulthood, men are on average 14 cm taller than women. This difference is almost entirely due to what happens at puberty – boys grow on average for two years longer after puberty, with an intense growth spurt occurring between the ages of fourteen and sixteen. Both sexes have a pubertal growth spurt of roughly six years, but girls reach maximum growth velocity early in puberty, about a year after the appearance of breast development. Boys don't reach their maximal height velocity until mid puberty. It is the combination of a longer growth period with a greater average yearly rate of growth that allows men to be taller than women.

During early puberty, limbs elongate first, leading to that funny coltish look of teenagers. Then the trunk begins to change, and then whoosh, suddenly they are beanpoles. When girls begin their periods, their growth slows down dramatically, with on average, only a further 5 cm of height being added. Because testosterone is such a potent anabolic steroid, boys acquire a dramatic increase in body mass index (BMI) from 16 to 21, almost all of which is down to the increase in the amount of lean tissue. The BMI of girls also increases, but in their case, the rise in BMI is largely down to an increase in body fat of about 11 kg. This might appear appalling to teenage girls, who seem to have a horror of fat, but it is the fat content of their bodies which determines their ability to have babies.

More growth hormone doesn't necessarily make you taller. You might think that all basketball players have hormone problems, since their average height now approaches 7'. Actually, they are simply constitutionally tall and have the same growth hormone levels as someone with constitutional short stature – what some people rather disparagingly call small normals. Excess growth hormone before a child has stopped growing is called gigantism. Excess growth hormone after growth has stopped, in adulthood, does not result in further height gain but in enlargement of the bones of jaw, hands and feet, a condition called acromegaly. One of the effects of growth hormone is on facial structure, turning the round soft faces of children into the more sculpted features of adults.

About one in 5,000 children is growth hormone deficient, with the condition being more common in boys than in girls – although this may simply be that small girls are less likely to be brought to a doctor's attention than small boys. There are many causes of deficiency, which include head injuries, tumours or radiotherapy affecting the pituitary gland. A child can be growth hormone deficient, or multiple-hormone deficient, lacking other hormones such as oestrogen or thyroid hormones. Certain medical conditions are also associated with short stature, such as chronic kidney disease, the chromosome disorder, Turner's Syndrome, and the genetic disease Prader Willi Syndrome in which short stature is also associated with obesity and learning difficulties.

Growth hormone used to be extracted, rather gruesomely, from pituitary glands collected from cadavers. There were always concerns about potential infection of those treated with cadaver-derived pituitary products and this was heightened even before the BSE crisis, when it became apparent that new variant Creutzfeldt Jakob disease (CJD) could be transmitted from one person to another through growth hormone preparations. The use of cadaver-derived products is now banned in most of Europe and in the US. For the last decade, all growth hormone has been produced using recombinant technology, which uses cells genetically engineered to secrete a particular product, a method of production now used for almost all hormones. It is safe, clean and provides hormones free from impurities. However, it is very costly indeed – about £20,000 for a year's treatment of one child. For 90 per cent of GH-deficient children, it increases rate of growth and increases final height to within the lower end of the normal range, preventing dwarfism (the fate of such children in the past).

Now, however, thanks to biotechnology, there is an unlimited, safe supply of growth hormone and the possibility of using GH to promote growth in non-growth hormone deficient short children has become a reality. To do this for those children with Turner's Syndrome or other non-GH medical problems affecting height is one thing, but there has been an increasing demand for growth hormone for normal healthy children, especially boys, who are just a bit short, especially for boys. What growth hormone won't do is make you grow beyond your height potential, so it may be of limited value, with a very small gain in height for rather too great a risk. Also, at what point do you decide that a child is likely to be short and when should you stop giving growth hormone? The answers are not clear, and nor are the side effects fully understood, yet one in five prescriptions for GH is still for 'idiopathic' height problems – in other words, for children that are healthy but destined to be smaller than average. In the US, there is even more pressure on physicians to prescribe GH. This is the first of many examples you will encounter in this book of hormones prescribed for lifestyle reasons.

So, there are three groups of hormone changes affecting teenagers: those to adrenal hormones, sex hormones and growth hormones. But there are also more subtle changes occurring in other hormone systems. For instance, the regulation of the stress hormone cortisol undergoes modifications during puberty. Cortisol stimulates the appetite and drives the extraordinary phenomenon that is teenage fridge-raiding and carbohydrate consumption. So far, though, I have not uncovered any research which indicates why they also consistently leave the empty packets behind them in the fridge. This is adaptive (the raiding, not the empty packets) in that fuel is required for growth and an increase in appetite ensures that they get it. There are also alterations in oxytocin, the hormone of bonding.

Teenage Behaviour

Teenagers get a rush from intensity, excitement and arousal: loud music, big dippers, horror movies, etc. In some teenagers this thrill-seeking and quest for novelty is subtle and easily managed. In others, their behaviour is more extreme and can get out of control. This is reflected in the statistics for teenage deaths, three quarters of which result from accident or misadventure.

Romeo and Juliet is the classic story of the way in which teenagers lose the ability to think logically or behave rationally. It is a story of adolescent love, in which passionate feelings accelerate at top speed and the motivation to be together transcends all else. Shakespeare gives Juliet's age as thirteen and the entire action, from first meeting to death, takes just four days. One day into their relationship, this girl and boy are already well on their way to spurning family, danger and public outrage, driven by emotional intensity. They act as if being together is more important than life itself. If they were adults, the psychiatrists would have had them sectioned by Day 2, never mind by Day 4.

It is tempting to believe – indeed, it has always been assumed – that such behaviour is entirely hormone driven. After all, aren't teenagers hormones on wheels? Having just read how hormones change during puberty, it does seem logical. However, links between hormone levels and poor behaviour in teenagers are either weak or non-existent. Certainly, high levels of hormones in teenage boys are not associated with emotional problems, and the evidence suggests that those with peak levels of sex hormones, whom you might expect to have the most emotional disturbance, are likely to be perfectly normal.

The changes that kick-start puberty – the release of gonado-trophin releasing hormone – begin in the brain, in the hypo-thalamus, which implies that the initial driver for the changes of puberty runs ahead of the hormonal system. Therefore it is likely to be the maturation of the brain that is behind the hormone level increases, and not the other way around.

It is particularly interesting to see the effects on the brain when hormones begin surging through the blood system. Hormones can directly affect only those brain cells which have the right receptors – for instance, neurons that produce the neurotransmitter sero-tonin (high levels of which result in feelings of calm and well-being) have oestrogen receptors, which means that rising levels of oestrogen have effects on mood and arousal via these receptors. There are also plenty of testosterone receptors in the brain too, meaning that the brain hears testosterone loud and clear and this affects behaviour.

A good example of the interactions between hormone and behaviour is seen in sleep. As every parent knows, teenagers find it very hard to get out of bed in the morning and to go to bed at night. Compare this with what they were like as five year olds, when you had trouble keeping them in bed beyond 6 in the morning. Actually this isn't just your teenagers being difficult, for a subtle biological shift in sleep patterns occurs during puberty. Once again, it's partly adaptive in that teenagers need more sleep for growth. There is an increased drive for sleepiness. But there is also an increase in the level of melatonin, the hormone of sleep, which is released only at night. One of the effects of this is similar to having gone through several time zones on a transatlantic flight. Hence the classic teen school-holiday pattern of sleeping from 2 a.m. until noon.

Come term time, the teenage body is in disarray as it is forced by a 7 a.m. wake-up call – while still on Planet MTV time – to gather itself together, even though it thinks it's 4 in the morning. These jet-lagged teenagers have come around by the end of the week to parental time zone hours, only to wreck themselves with another bout of 2 a.m. to noon sleeping at the weekend. Many become chronically sleep deprived, with all the implications for behaviour that that implies – irritability, unable to concentrate, with poor attention span – which are inevitably reflected in their school performance.

Parents are not much help here. Urging their offspring to go to bed means that they go to their rooms at bedtime only to surf the net, text their mates and watch late-night TV because they find it impossible to sleep – just as we adults would if we were jet-lagged. So the hormone involvement is relatively modest; it is the knock-on effect of changes in behaviour that wreak the havoc.

Teenagers and Sex

The behaviour that is entirely hormone-driven in teenage boys is their sexual appetite. They go from thinking girls are silly, soppy creatures in pink, to being completely girl-obsessed. It is said that teenage boys think about sex every seven seconds. As little as that? For boys, adolescence is one long wankfest. Teenagers can ejaculate and have another erection barely minutes later. Compare this to men in their fifties, where the recovery time, or refractory period (as it is called), may be several hours. For teenage boys the mere sight of a woman is enough to engender an erection, whereas forty years on it will require manual stimulation of the penis to prompt an erection, no matter how erotic the situation. As puberty brings more testosterone with every new dawn, so boys become ever more sexually rampant. In early puberty they are puny, smaller than girls and rather unattractive to them. Their greatest hope of actually finding a girl that is willing (in their dreams), lies not in their testosterone-supercharged sex drive, which girls in general find rather unattractive in its lack of subtlety, but in the changes that testosterone makes to their bodies, in fashioning a broader, more muscular, leaner adult from the body of a child. It takes several years for boys to learn to live with their testosterone, and gradually those inappropriately timed erections and sexual obsessions begin to calm down.

This period of rampant hormones but still puny bodies is an important learning period. In general, teenage boys of this age are roundly rejected by girls, despite their boasts to each other, but one day those carefully honed chat-up lines will have the desired effect.

Oestrogen is only one of the hormones involved in sexual response in women, as we saw in the previous chapter, and human females are covert about their sexuality, not advertising when they are fertile. Girls are not therefore as overwhelmed by their sexuality as boys. Nevertheless they are beginning to preen and become sexual beings. This can be very disturbing if they are younger than the age at which society considers sexual activity acceptable, and it is also a cause for alarm, for their brain is still that of a child, with a marked immaturity and specifically an inability to understand the consequences of risk.

Baby Adults or Adult Babies?

The thing that is really irritating about teenagers (and by now you will have guessed that I have two teenage boys) is that one moment their behaviour is that of adults, while the next it is that of a not-very-bright three year old, or possibly, a retarded chimp. Or an amoeba. Going from captaining a rugby side, for instance, where their increased strength and agility, not to mention mature social skills, are fully deployed, to kicking a rugby ball in the sitting room . . . and being astonished when their mother goes into orbit because the ball has just smashed a picture. The rapid oscillation between child and adult is one of the hallmarks of the teenager.

In fact teenage brains are going through a process of maturation and it is this maturation which many now believe is responsible for much of the behaviour that we classically attribute to hormones. These changes are actually entirely independent of hormones and are a function of age, which is illustrated by those children who, for various medical reasons, do not go through puberty and yet are cognitively normal.

It has been discovered only very recently that there are two main features of brain maturation that happen to coincide with puberty. Previously it was believed that the brain was pretty well set by adolescence but in the last couple of years, and to everyone's surprise, it has been realized that maturation is not completed until late teens or even early twenties. One feature is that myelin, a sort of fatty insulating material, is added to axons, the main transmission lines of the nervous system, which has the effect of speeding up messages. The other feature is a pruning of nerve connections, the synapses, in the pre-frontal cortex. This area of the brain is responsible for what is called executive action, which is a shopping list of the things that teenagers lack – such as goal-setting, priority-setting, planning, organization and impulse-inhibition. During childhood, for reasons that are not clear, a tangle of nerve cells sprout in this brain area, which lies behind the eyes, but during puberty these areas of increased synaptic density are then reduced by about half, presumably to increase efficiency.

These changes in the adolescent brain primarily affect motivation and emotion, which manifest themselves as mood swings, conflict with authority and risk-taking. For example, it is not just testosterone that drives risk-taking, but the inability of the immature brain to assess risk properly that gets teenagers into trouble.

The remodelling of the cortex helps explain another feature of teenagers: their astonishing level of self-centredness. For a while, as their brain is undergoing changes, they find it hard to recognize other people's emotions. This has been demonstrated in a number of research studies: if you show teenagers pictures of faces, they will be some 20 per cent less accurate in gauging the emotions depicted, and don't re-acquire this ability until they are eighteen or so. This makes them socially inept, unable to read social situations – or in parental language, a nightmare. They seem unable to read the signs, are unaware when they are treading on thin ice with their behaviour, and furthermore have no appreciation of parental feelings or of the impact of what they are doing on those around them. Teenagers exist in a universe of one.

It has nothing to do with hormones, but let me say a word about addiction. One of the reasons why we get hooked on tobacco for example, is that we tried it as an adolescent. The teenage brain gets a bigger bang from nicotine than an adult one does. The same is true of alcohol and drugs too. This intense reward increases the likelihood of addiction. Indeed, one of the strongest predictors of alcoholism is the age of first initiation. It's a deadly combination – increased likelihood of addiction coupled with poor assessment of risk.

Testosterone (Again)

Research shows that the No. 1 risk factor in homicide is maleness, and the second is youth. Teenage boys are primarily the violent ones, rather than girls. Boys have testosterone, girls don't. Surely this must implicate testosterone as a cause of violence?

First, there is no consistent relationship between normal circulating testosterone levels and violence in teenagers. In fact some studies have shown a negative association. You could turn the question around and ask whether testosterone levels are linked to popularity and respect by peers in teenagers. I suspect there would be a greater likelihood of finding such a correlation as many studies have shown high levels of testosterone and leadership to be linked.

Being split up from your best mate is a peril of adolescence. 'They're a bad influence on you' is the general gist of parental or teacher wisdom on this one. Actually, one hypothesis is that teenage boys pick up cues from the environment and use them to determine 'normal' behaviour. This is illustrated by recent work from the Medical Research Council (MRC) unit at the Institute of Psychiatry, which shows that it is not testosterone levels that determine your waywardness as a teenager but the people you hang with. Keep the company of bad boys and you will take your behaviour cue from them. Hang out with sober sorts and your behaviour will be like theirs. Testosterone levels are related to leadership in boys with non-deviant peers and to aggression in those with deviant mates. I say this despite the ignominy of proving Mrs Glass, form teacher of Year 9, right.

What boys are concerned with, if not always consciously, is status. Much of the driver for male behaviour is that women, with whom teenage boys are obsessed, find power and status irresistible in a man. Lower status men find themselves ignored by women who consistently prefer partners who can impress them. So impress they must if they are to secure their ideal woman. On one level, this is classic boy meets girl stuff, but make no mistake it is underpinned by a specific and very powerful biological drive, for the right choice of mate is essential if you are to transmit your genes to the next generation.

If levels of testosterone are not closely linked to teenage violence, what is? Deprivation in childhood. The theory – and there is a wealth of literature on this subject – is that if low status males are to avoid the road to genetic nothingness (the words of neuroscientist Steven Pinker), they may have to adopt aggressive, high-risk strategies. If you've got nothing, you have nothing to lose through your behaviour. Certainly in humans, both violence and risk-taking behaviour show a pronounced social gradient, being lowest in the highest social classes and highest in the lowest ones. This is surely not what you would expect if testosterone were the only driver of violence.

Respect is everything in deprived communities and a great deal of violence is initiated by perceived slights to status. As Sir Michael Marmot, the distinguished epidemiologist, points out in his book *The Status Syndrome*, we are shaped by evolution to seek status. Professors don't kill each other when jockeying for position in being given grants, although they frequently knife with words and bludgeon with faint praise in a poisonously competitive atmosphere – and in any case, the law is rather touchy about murder. But if you are at the bottom of the heap, with every chance of spending time in prison, with those closest to you living fractured, short lives, and with no chance of taking a place in mainstream society, how long are you likely to spend in weighing up the result of your actions before lashing out, or even murdering someone? How much more likely, then, is this to be the case for teenagers, as adolescence is the period in life when the brain's ability to fully consider the implications of action is seriously compromised?

The hormone link to high-risk choices is likely not to be testosterone, at least not initially, but the stress hormone cortisol. Stress during early life raises cortisol levels, so increasing behavioural problems (such as hyperactivity). These tend to make children more aggressive, less affiliative and more likely to perceive others as threatening. Stress either in pregnancy or in early life permanently resets the stress response of the child, so that there is an increased reaction to stress – known as hyperarousal. A stressed child, when meeting someone new (even in a familiar environment), will withdraw and refuse to make eye contact, rather than chat happily. This increased stress response plays out in reduced life expectancy because cortisol affects almost every body system. It is also closely linked with depressive illness.

So testosterone plays a part here only after the fact. Aggression and stress raise testosterone levels. Aggression and stress also reinforce each other at the biological level. Animal work reported in the journal *Behavioural Neuroscience* in October 2004 suggests that there is a fast feedback loop between stress hormones and the hypothalamus, which allows aggressive behaviour to escalate.

Testosterone in Adults

Let me digress briefly from the teenage years. Whilst testosterone is not necessarily a marker for violent behaviour in teenagers, in adulthood, high testosterone levels are strongly linked to criminality, with those committing the most violent crimes, and especially the ones that cause most trouble and confrontation within prison, tending to be those that have the highest testosterone levels.

Testosterone in humans is about dominance, not aggression: most men assert their dominance without recourse to violence. For instance, in a series of studies examining the links between testosterone and brief social encounters, people with high testosterone displayed a more forward and businesslike manner, and were those people most likely to impress on first encounter. Lock men away in a closed environment, and the one that is most dominant is likely to have the highest testosterone level. In fact anti-social acts are often not violent, but just attempts to dominate figures of authority (teachers, policemen etc).

Testosterone levels also alter with stress. Professor James Dabbs of Georgia State University is the leading authority in this field, and has focused his research on male children and adults, lawyers and criminals, sportsmen and even politicians using saliva to test testosterone levels. His work on sportsmen is particularly interesting. For two hours after a competition, testosterone levels in the winners are elevated, while those of the losers are reduced. If the winner feels that he was lucky or didn't really deserve to win, the rise in testosterone is less marked. During a study of football fans who watched Brazil beat Italy in the 1994 World Cup, testosterone was increased significantly post-match in Brazilian fans. Guess who won the match? The point is that testosterone levels rise and fall with experience of success or failure and even with anticipation of those things. In general, testosterone rises following aggression but is not a cause of aggression per se.

Dabbs also studied some women prisoners, showing that high testosterone levels are related to criminal violence and aggressive dominance, rather than being a uniquely male hormone. In the next chapter, we will see that women have testosterone too – quite a bit of it.

Hormone Determinism

Professor Dabbs claims that innate levels of testosterone can predict your future effectively. White-collar workers have lower testosterone than blue-collar workers; actors and football players have higher levels than vicars. This opens up a number of possibilities: could teenagers be tested and then steered towards those professions most suited to their testosterone levels – or could those with lower levels even be given supplements? To be honest, I'm not that convinced by this work, which seems like hormone determinism to me. Hormones are just part of what you are and there's more to human life than the endocrine system, magnificent though it is.

Stress and Depression

Major depression often becomes apparent for the first time in adolescence. Although it may be triggered by a life event (bereavement, family break-up) it is more likely to happen to those who are already genetically susceptible. Depression is twice as likely in teenage girls than in boys, a pattern which will endure for life. This poses the question, could it be attributed to the ovarian steroids unleashed in puberty?

During adolescence, reproductive hormones make girls more sensitive to the effects of stress. In addition, this occurs at a time when the stress response is changing, with more cortisol being produced. Although the basic level of cortisol secretion does not vary across the menstrual cycle, women become more sensitive to it, particularly during the luteal phase, which is the second, post-ovulation, half of their cycle. As I explain elsewhere, high levels of cortisol are a feature of depressive illness. Many researchers suggest that society's view of women affects self-esteem and creates feelings of worthlessness, which is why more women have depress-ive illness. I'm not convinced by this as a reason for this high rate of depression in women. Since sex hormones have an effect on mood when women are on the pill, when they are taking the progestogen element of HRT and in the second half of their cycle, a biological explanation seems rather more plausible, with hormones the most likely culprits.

Puberty

In the UK, 95 per cent of girls will have menstruated by fifteen, and 50 per cent by the age of twelve and a half. The age at which normal puberty occurs is heavily influenced by genes. If your mother started her periods early, probably you will too. Ethnicity is also important – with blacks starting before whites, and whites before Asians, as a vastly generalized rule. Periods are actually quite a late event of puberty in girls, but their start (called the menarche) is a convenient and well-defined marker, which is often used as an indicator of puberty, even though the process has actually begun some years before. Environment is also very influential. If you have experienced serious illness as a small child, or you have been very short of food, puberty will be delayed. Extra hormones are not necessarily required in these situations. A team from Israel found recently that supplementing a child's diet, particularly with Vitamin A and iron, was as effective as hormonal therapy.

What is the trigger for puberty? In girls, it is associated with a critical body mass, or rather a critical percentage of body fat. And when leptin, a hormone that is produced by fat, was discovered a decade ago, everyone thought that they had discovered the puberty 'on' switch. Certainly, children (boys and girls) who have no leptin because of a rare gene defect do not go through puberty, but will do so if given leptin. There is a gender difference in leptin secretion: it rises throughout puberty in girls, but not in boys. However, since fat mass steadily increases during this time in girls (and decreases in boys) and leptin is produced by fat, this isn't surprising. Leptin and the initiation of puberty is the subject of intense study at the moment, but early indications are that it is not *the* 'on' trigger as was originally thought. Instead it is thought to have a permissive role. In other words, when the noise from leptin is loud enough, something, previously held in check, is allowed to happen, which then cranks up the hypothalamus to let loose the gonadotrophin releasing hormone. Whatever the trigger, which could well be initiated in the brain itself, as suggested earlier, the hypothalamus goes through a change – from not responding to oestrogen with a surge of luteinising hormone which will prompt ovulation, to doing precisely that.

IS PUBERTY GETTING EARLIER?

Over the last century, the age at first period has dramatically decreased. It is likely that menarche for girls in the nineteenth century was around seventeen because of poor health and nutritional factors, such as, crucially, lack of access to fresh foods in winter. Victorian novels are full of young girls complaining of 'green sickness' or 'chlorosis'. Today we would call this iron-deficient anaemia and lack of iron is one of the factors that can help delay puberty. Between the mid-nineteenth and the mid-twentieth century, age at first period went down from seventeen to fourteen in the US and the better developed European countries. Today, US figures are 12.9 in white Americans and 12.7 in black Americans. Across the world today, the average age at menarche varies enormously, with those girls living in underprivileged conditions in China and Senegal (two countries where studies have been carried out) still experiencing their first period at an average age of sixteen. Interestingly, there is a North–South gradient, which has existed for at least a century, with higher ages at menarche in Scandinavia, for example, than in France. The trend towards lower menarche seems to have bottomed out with Britain, Sweden and Belgium seeing a small increase in menarchal age, while it is still declining in Denmark, France and Finland.

One of the problems of these statistics is the different markers that are used to express age at puberty. I have already mentioned age at first period, which is a relatively late indicator, but another, which is frequently used, is B2 or thelarche, which describes when breast development first appears. This precedes menarche and is not always easy to assess, particularly in children who are obese, and there is quite a variation between assessors' estimates – something which makes you suspicious about the reliability of the data. This age seems to be diminishing fairly dramatically in the US, and is now 8.4 for white girls and 9.5 in black Americans. There is no such trend in Europe. Precocious puberty is defined in Europe as less than eight, for breast development and less than nine for the parallel testicular development in boys. But in the US, the age limit has now been reset to under seven in Caucasian girls and six in African Americans – for breast development. Onset of periods seems to have halted at an older age and is showing no sign of further decrease. What is interesting is that the time between onset of periods and regular cycling seems to be increasing, from 1.9 to three years.

Precocious puberty is twenty times more common in girls than in boys, and in 90 per cent of them there is no obvious cause. In boys, less than 10 per cent of cases have no identifiable cause and most have some underlying problem such as pituitary tumours. There is also a phenomenon in which children adopted from developing countries and then raised in a more affluent environment have an increased incidence of early puberty. In a study from Belgium, there was an eighty-fold increase in incidence of sexual precocity in children adopted from abroad, compared to native Belgian children. It is surprising, however, that no such reports come from the US, where physicians are as attuned to the problem, and where over 100,000 children have been adopted, over the last decade, often from very deprived circumstances.

Diets that have a high fat rather than high vegetable matter content are associated with early onset of periods, and diets high in phytoestrogens (natural oestrogen-like chemicals found in plants) with a later onset. This might be especially relevant for children adopted from deprived countries where plant oestrogens are a large part of the diet. There has also been a big decrease in the amount of exercise taken by children over the last fifty years: those in developed countries are more likely to be in front of the TV than out exercising. Increasing fat levels may be sending out a louder leptin signal, earlier than before, as a result, while those in developing countries may be involved in hard physical work by puberty, which is likely to decrease their body fat. It seems highly likely then that early puberty is the result of lifestyle factors, although this is not the view of some activists who feel that early puberty reflects exposure to ubiquitous chemicals in the modern environment.

DECREASING AGE OF PUBERTY – AN EFFECT OF CHEMICALS?

Although precocious puberty in girls is widespread in the USA, particularly among African Americans, there is no such phenomenon in western Europe. There is no suggestion that boys are affected either, in the US or in Europe. You would also expect – if there really was a problem caused by chemicals – there to be disturbance of other secondary sexual characteristics, such as inappropriate body hair or disturbances of growth, particularly those affecting the timing of the changes seen in the growing zone at the ends of long bones, which signal the end of growth. These have not been seen. In the Belgian study of children adopted from abroad, it is suggested that the children, who all had detectable levels of DDT, were exposed to it in their home country, and that it exerted an inhibitory effect on the pituitary, and that interrupted exposure caused precocious puberty on emigration. This seems to me like a conclusion looking for data which simply isn't there. DDT is still used to control mosquitoes in some developing countries, where death from malaria is common and feared, and it would be a surprise if residues were not found in children. But to call the DDT causal is stretching the evidence. If this is truly the case, it is odd that a similar effect hasn't been found amongst the 100,000 children adopted into the USA from other countries over the last decade, or indeed in Britain. The major changes in nutrition, lifestyle and body fat are much more likely to be the cause than endocrine disrupting chemicals.

Teenage Genius

This chapter has contained a rather gloomy picture of the adolescent brain. Can I redress the balance and close by saying that teenagers are also our salvation. Their brains are more open to ideas, they are more amenable to change and are less set in their ways because they come without the baggage of experience that binds creative thought so tightly. I don't think it is an accident that teenagers are behind some of the world's great discoveries, particularly in technology. An example of what I mean is Ada, Countess of Lovelace, muse to Charles Babbage, he of the difference engine and father of computing. It was seventeen-year-old Ada, the daughter of the poet Lord Byron, who saw the potential of Babbage's invention, predicting that it could be used to manipulate figures and symbols. That's a teenager's insight for you.

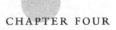

CHAPTER FOUR

HORMONES AND THE ENVIRONMENT

The last chapter closed with an account of the fall in the age at which puberty occurs. This chapter is about chemicals, natural and synthetic, which have hormone-like actions and are found in the environment around us, in water, air and food, and indeed, in the very fabric of our daily lives, in cosmetics, plastics and household chemicals. Many believe that these hormones are responsible not only for the fall in the age of puberty, but for falling sperm counts, increased incidence of testicular cancers and other male reproductive abnormalities plus higher rates of breast cancer and fertility problems in women. This is an evolving story, in which I would not presume to lay claim to the truth, for it has not yet been fully revealed. What I can do is give you perspective and sanity.

Gender Bender Chemicals

Endocrine disruptors are chemicals, both natural and man-made, which mimic, block or otherwise disrupt the action of human hormones. Also called gender benders, they are the subject of considerable concern and this is reflected in the proposed European Union (EU) chemicals legislation known as REACH (Regulation, Evaluation and Authorization of Chemicals). All new chemicals are strictly evaluated and tested for toxicity, but those produced prior to 1981 have 'squatter's rights' and, until now, have not been subject to current testing regimes. This is about to change and some 30,000 chemicals will now have to undergo a range of safety tests, to check whether they cause endocrine disruption – as single compounds or in combination with other substances. Clearly, chemicals can have a different effect when combined, so this is an important development, although one wonders whether anyone has done the maths here. The number of combinations possible with 30,000 different chemicals is greater than the number of atoms in the universe. Another problem is that there is as yet no universally agreed testing procedure to identify endocrine disruptors. Some scientists, such as Fred Vom Saal, Professor of Biological Sciences at the University of Missouri, famously claim that normal dose response testing (in which you increase the dose until you see an effect) is not appropriate for these compounds, which he believes are more toxic in tiny quantities than in larger ones.

This is a hugely contentious area, and one which polarizes opinion. There is a steamroller common-sense logic to many of the media headlines, and indeed popular perception. For instance, early puberty is thought to be 'unnatural' and therefore it stands to reason that there must be an 'unnatural' cause for this phenomenon. Man-made endocrine disruptors fit the bill in a way that sedentary fat kids do not.

There are many chemicals that are extremely hazardous – toxic – in large amounts, with direct exposure. Farmers that mix crop sprays themselves are likely to be far more acutely exposed, for instance, than the people who eventually eat the cabbages that were sprayed. Some chemicals are banned altogether, either because of their high toxicity, or because of evidence of bioaccumulation (that is, they are not excreted but sequestered by the body, usually into fat, and because they may also 'bioconcentrate', that is become more concentrated the further up the food chain an animal is) or because they are persistent, remaining in the environment for many years. The pesticide DDT, which has been banned in many countries for over thirty years, is all three, being toxic, bioaccumulative *and* persistent. Similarly PCBs (polychlorinated biphenyls), which are mixtures of chlorinated compounds used in coolants, lubricants and in electrical devices, are all three: toxic, bioaccumulative and persistent. They too are now banned. In both Europe and the US, pesticides are highly regulated and their levels in the environment have been steadily falling over the last decade.

There is now greater concern about those chemicals which are ubiquitous in our lives, for instance bisphenol A (a polymer used to line food tins and generally in plastics) phthalates (used as a softener in plastics), flame retardants and many of the chemicals found in toiletries and cosmetics. The common thread linking all these chemicals is their ability to alter hormone action in the body. They have weak hormonal or anti-hormonal activity, usually oestrogenic (behaving like female hormones), androgenic (behaving like male hormones) or anti-androgenic or anti-oestrogenic. Some substances have combinations of effect depending on the dose and may indeed be beneficial in small doses – an effect called hormesis – while being harmful at higher concentrations. They may also have great, or no, effect, depending on the stage of life at which an organism is exposed to them. Thus endocrine disruptors are more likely to result in harmful effects if exposure takes place during fetal development than in old age.

Before you rush off screaming, let's put this in context. We eat large quantities of foods every day which have endocrine-disrupting activity – in fact, almost every mouthful contains something with hormone-altering ability – without harm. Plant foods contain at least 12,000 chemicals which they produce for structural, attractant, chemoprotective and hormonal purposes. For instance, cabbage contains forty-nine natural pesticides, some of which are banned for use by farmers because they can cause cancer in laboratory rats. Eating cabbage – and indeed other members of the cabbage family like cauliflower and turnips – will affect the function of the thyroid as well as inhibit the action of oestrogen. Most beans, such as soy beans and chick peas, contain chemicals called isoflavones which have both oestrogenic and anti-oestrogenic activity. Plant chemicals which affect human oestrogen levels are called phytoestrogens and are discussed at greater length in Chapter 6 in relation to alleviating the symptoms of menopause. Such foods have been part of the human diet for centuries and common sense suggests that we need not fear them. Certainly no one would think twice about the hormone-disrupting effect of coleslaw before eating it.

What has fuelled the media anxiety, however, is the well-documented 'feminization of nature', the phenomenon of man-made endocrine disruptors causing problems in aquatic wildlife. It was a story that started some fifteen years ago, when it was noticed that the male alligators in Lake Apopka, Florida, had abnormally small testicles and low testosterone levels. It was thought that it could have been caused by the oestrogenic effects of the pesticide DDT and its breakdown product, DDE. Breakdown products of the PCBs present in the lake were also known to act as synthetic oestrogens following experiments with turtle eggs. Depending on temperature, crocodile and turtle eggs are either predominately male or female. If these eggs are incubated at a 'male' temperature, but painted with PCBs, sex reversal occurs, just as if the egg had been painted with oestrogen. A disturbing number of similar effects on wildlife were noted, principally amongst aquatic animals but also amongst panthers and other major carnivores.

Another, very dramatic example of an endocrine disruptor is TBT (tributyltin), which is an anti-fouling agent painted on to ships' hulls. It leaches into seawater where it masculinizes female shellfish, preventing reproduction. This chemical will be banned by 2008. TBT isn't oestrogenic but it still has a gender-bending effect, pushing up testosterone levels in female shellfish.

Observation of fish from sewage treatment water lagoons in England and Wales has indicated that many possess both male and female features. This caused alarm and a series of tests using a vitellogenin assay were instituted. This is a substance produced normally by female fish which is under the control of oestrogens. Males don't produce it unless exposed to high doses of oestrogen, so it is frequently used as a test of environmental oestrogen presence.

Rainbow trout that had been exposed to sewage treatment water showed a 100,000–500,000-fold increase in plasma vitellogenin concentrations and male fish had levels almost as high as females. More recently, the Environment Agency, the environmental regulator in Britain, published a report in 2004 that showed that of 1,500 fish at fifty river sites, more than a third of males displayed female characteristics, with young fish especially vulnerable. The effects seemed to worsen with increased exposure. There is a wealth of other data confirming the widespread wildlife effects of endocrine-disrupting chemicals.

Some scientists claim that similar effects can occur in humans. In 1993, two scientists, Richard Sharpe and Niels Skakkebaek, put forward the hypothesis that increased oestrogen exposure in early life increases the risk of two specific genital malformations in humans: hypospadias, where the urethral opening does not appear at the tip of the penis, and cryptorchidism (in which the testicles don't descend properly), together with those of testicular cancer and lowered sperm count (these conditions together are called testicular dysgenesis syndrome). The origins of all these abnormalities are thought to arise in fetal life when the male reproductive tract is being formed. Supporting evidence for this theory came from boys exposed to the potent synthetic oestrogen DES during their mother's pregnancy, among whom such abnormalities were more common. Rising rates of these problems were soon being suggested as proof of endocrine disruption in humans.

All these issues received far greater prominence in 1996 with the publication of American journalist Theo Colborn's book, *Our Stolen Future*, which has had a similar impact to that of *Silent Spring*, Rachel Carson's book about pesticides two decades earlier. In 1996, an influential multi award-winning film was screened on BBC television: *Horizon*'s '*Assault on the male*'.

So what is the evidence for the effects on humans? The deterioration in male reproductive health over the last two decades has been marked in some ways, but very patchy. Sperm counts are said to have declined, but there is enormous regional variation. In the world sperm league, Finns seem to have very high counts, as do New Yorkers, while Denmark and the inhabitants of other American cities, such as San Francisco, lurk near the bottom of the table. Sperm count is also extremely variable within the same man – let alone between men – and is affected by a huge range of factors from sedentary occupations (which far more men have now than in the past) to amount of sexual activity. In fact, abstinence is the single biggest confounding variable for both sperm count and quality. It is literally a case of 'use it or lose it', as the more sperm that is used, the more sperm is produced in response. If a man does not ejaculate regularly, sperm quality and quantity quickly falls. Of particular concern in comparisons of sperm counts is that methods of appraising quality have changed considerably over the last thirty years, making true comparisons difficult.

There is no doubt that testicular cancer rates have increased, with a trebling of rates in some countries not uncommon, and the disease now appears in younger men. In Britain, the incidence of this uncommon cancer has doubled over the last thirty years. Again the data, although much more solid than that relating to sperm count, varies by country. Denmark has the highest incidence of testicular cancer, whereas nearby Finland has one of the lowest rates. The rise in this cancer pre-dates the introduction of many of the chemicals under suspicion, and whilst levels of many of these are now falling, the rate still appears to be increasing. The rates first started to rise in Britain in the 1920s, so if we are talking of effects on the fetus being causative, we must be speaking of an era prior to 1900.

Aside from the food we eat, where have these oestrogens come from? It used to be something of an urban myth that women on the pill were changing the sex of fish in the Thames. Now it is known to be scientific fact.

Oestrogens – There's A Lot of Them About

Humans, of both sexes, excrete oestrogens in both faeces and urine. Animals do too. Oestrogens come in several varieties, but the main ones of interest here are, in rising order of potency, oestriol, oestrone and oestradiol. Although oestrogens are largely excreted in the form of inactive complexes, some decoupling of these complexes seems to occur during sewage treatment, which restores activity.

Men excrete up to 3.9 microgrammes (μg) of oestrone per day in their urine. Compare this with menopausal women who excrete up to 5.6 μg per day, or up to 33 μg per day in those on HRT. Women in the second half of their cycle account for 11.7 μg per day and those who are pregnant excrete a phenomenal 550 μg per day, in both urine and faeces.

Oestradiol is the most potent natural oestrogen. In urine and faeces, menstruating women excrete up to 4.6 μg per day and pregnant women up to 445 μg per day. Men, by the way, excrete up to 2.4 μg per day of this hormone.

But it is ethinyloestradiol – the synthetic oestrogen in the pill – which is of special concern as it is twenty-five times more potent than natural oestradiol. Women taking the pill excrete on average 10.5 μg per day, which is about 40 per cent of the 26 μg taken each day in their pill. Most of it is in their urine. To get a better idea of potency, you'd need to take 4 mg of the natural oestradiol a day to have the same contraceptive effect as just 50 μg per day of the synthetic version. The synthetic sort is used in the pill because it is not broken down as quickly in blood, so ensuring its continuing contraceptive effect.

Overall, every adult in Britain is excreting on average 10.5 μg per day of oestrone and 6.6 μg per day of oestradiol. By far and away the biggest natural oestrogen polluters are pregnant women. Add to this the run-off from animals' urine and faeces, and you've got a huge natural source of oestrogen pollution which was clearly around long before the advent of the pill. However, it is estimated that around 80 per cent of oestradiol, 65 per cent of oestrone and 85 per cent of the synthetic oestradiol are removed during water treatment in activated sludge plants.

Despite the fact that synthetic oestradiol is at the only just detectable limit in water, steroid oestrogens are still the most potent endocrine disruptor found in sewage effluent. One clue that they are causing problems in water is that intersex roach are found mainly downstream of sewage effluent outfalls, not upstream of them. One wonders – had anyone investigated thirty years ago – whether there would have been as many intersex fish then as now? For in the 1960s and 1970s, when many women took the pill, the dosage of synthetic oestrogen was much, much higher than it is now. But back in the 1960s, pollution – and thus oxygen depletion – was so great in our rivers,that people were simply counting dead fish rather than looking to see whether they had breeding abnormalities.

There is another source of natural exposure to oestrogens. Mammals are adapted to starting life inside their mothers, whose bloodstreams are rich in oestrogens. Maternal and fetal blood does not mix, however, and despite the fetal adrenal glands being steroid factories, the baby is not directly exposed to them for they are passed over to the placenta in a semi-constructed, less active form. However, although many of the sex steroids in amniotic fluid are bound to a chemical called alphafetoprotein or AFP (which you may know better as the basis of the test for spina bifida), the fluid is still a pond, highly enriched with potent female sex steroids, which babies sit and swallow in, suggesting that babies, in particular boys, have some defence against their feminizing effects. As we saw in Chapter 2, hormones effectively decide the sex of boys, for even if their chromosomes say 'male', without a rush of male hormones being switched on at the crucial point in pregnancy, a chromosomally male child will appear to be female. The default sex in the womb is female, until the Y chromosome switches on production of testosterone.

There is some evidence that variations in the concentration of maternal oestrogen are associated with an increased risk of testicular cancer and cryptorchidism in boys, and it has been suggested that today's high-fat low-fibre diet, which increases maternal circulating oestrogen, could be responsible for both these effects in boys and increased breast cancer rates. Also of interest is that testicular abnormalities are more likely in first-born children who are boys. Oestrogen levels are highest in first pregnancies.

OESTROGENIC CHEMICALS

Those pesticides that have oestrogenic activity, such as PCBs, are now banned. Banned too is the use of DES, a synthetic oestrogen used to prevent miscarriage in the 1950s and 1960s. However, many of the chemicals that are used ubiquitously such as bisphenol A and phthalates, also have an oestrogenic, or anti-oestrogenic action. Bisphenol A, which was originally developed by chemists as a synthetic oestrogen before finding wider use in plastics, binds to the oestrogen receptor in order to persuade cells that this is a genuine message from oestrogen. Phthalates, which were banned in children's toys and childcare products in Europe in 2004, prevent natural oestrogen binding to its own receptor.

These chemicals are everywhere – we can't just take them out of the environment. Nor would we find life very comfortable or convenient without them. Although these particular chemicals – phthalates and bisphenols – are individually five orders of magnitude (100,000) times less potent than the oestrogen in your own body, and a hundredfold less potent than the phytoestrogens found in food which you eat all the time. There is a concern about additionality, which means that small doses of many different chemicals may amplify their effect more than the sum of the individual chemicals. Given all this, it is hardly surprising that some scientists believe that, just like fish, humans live in a sea of oestrogens, which is reflected in rising rates not just of these male reproductive effects, but also of breast cancer.

BREAST CANCER

People think that because breast cancer rates have risen so rapidly that there must be an environmental cause for it. We know that breast cancer is largely a hormone-driven cancer, with about 75 per cent of tumours having oestrogen receptors. The greatest risk of breast cancer is age (there's much more on this in Chapter 6) and many of the other risk factors concern your body's lifetime exposure to your own oestrogen. For instance, the longer the time between the start of periods and the menopause, the higher the risk; the fatter you are the greater the risk, because being fat is associated with higher levels of circulating oestrogens, and so on. Great changes in lifestyle account for some of the increased incidence: women start their periods earlier and have fewer babies at a later age than they did a generation ago; they are also fatter and drink more alcohol, all factors known to increase risk. Some of the rise can be put down to to the introduction of breast cancer screening – there was a noticeably increased 'blip' in cases when regular screening started in Britain. Taking all these factors into account there is thought to be a true rise in incidence of about 5 per cent, for reasons that are unknown. It might be chemicals. It could be lifestyle or something else completely, but it is easier to lay the blame on chemicals, because this is something we feel we can control by campaigning and regulation.

Breast cancer is a disease that can develop and progress over a woman's entire life but it is thought that puberty is the time when young girls are at greatest risk of potential damage by cancer-causing agents. So could exposure to oestrogen mimics in adolescence be the cause of today's high rates of breast cancer? One study linked exposure to organochlorine chemicals, which are oestrogenic and accumulate in breast fat, to breast cancer but most subsequent studies have not confirmed this. For many years, synthetic oestrogens in the pill were associated with increased rates of breast cancer. Now it is known that although breast cancer risk is increased slightly while taking the pill, there is no long-term effect. There is an effect on breast cancer incidence for those taking HRT for five years or more, which is equivalent to that of drinking two glasses of wine a day. The general consensus seems to be that in the causation of breast cancer, endocrine disruptors are much less likely to be as important compared to a woman's own hormones.

The most confusing aspect of the debate about endocrine disruptors is that on the one hand there is concern about synthetic oestrogenic chemicals causing breast cancer, but on the other, women are being urged to eat more of the foods that contain phyto-estrogens in order to *prevent* breast cancer, because it is seen that women who consume large quantities in the Far East have the lowest rates of this disease. This does seem very contradictory. Is it simply that synthetic oestrogens are potent and bad, whereas natural oestrogens are weak and good, promoting positive rather than negative health benefits? A recent piece of research, in which a range of types of oestrogens were introduced to an immature mouse womb, showed that once they interacted with the oestrogen receptors in the tissue, a natural oestrogen, genistein (a phyto-estrogen) and a synthetic oestrogen each switched on exactly the same 179 genes within the cell. Thus, at a cellular level, no distinction is made between man-made plant and natural forms of oestrogen. Each has risks and benefits depending on the tissue targeted and the time of the exposure. None are all good or all bad.

Another very specific breast cancer scare related to parabens, which have oestrogenic activity and are found in many cosmetics and body products. Parabens are said to be the cause of rising breast cancer levels because of their use in deodorants, particularly by children. The first thing you need to know is that most underarm products do not contain parabens. This is not because spooked manufacturers have suddenly removed them. This has always been the case, because the normal preservative for deodorant is alcohol. Parabens – usually added as as a preservative – are not needed. Aside from this minor point, those who say underarm products and breast cancer are linked point to the way rising sales mirror the rising incidence of breast cancer. Saying that there is a correlation is a bit like linking postwar sales of bananas and birth rates. True, these did rise together, but do bananas beget babies? If underarm products really were the cause of breast cancer, you'd see cause before effect – a big rise in product sales followed (since cancer takes decades to develop) years later by a corresponding rise in breast cancer incidence. That's not the picture we are presented with. You'd also expect there to be more breast cancer in countries with high anti-perspirant/deodorant use. Japan and America have markedly different rates of breast cancer but the same use of deodorants. Worry about something else.

Anti-Androgenic Effects

If there are rising rates of conditions causing male infertility, then it would make more sense for these conditions to be caused by substances with an anti-androgenic effect, which would affect the amount of testosterone produced. There are now many chemicals which are anti-androgens, although these substances, which have been introduced since the Second World War, cannot explain the early rise in testicular cancer.

Male rats exposed to phthalates – plasticizers, some of which can have an anti-androgen effect – have low rates of fertility and a higher risk of developing a testicular cancer. Phthalates can build up in the body, with women at reproductive age seeming to have higher levels than the rest of the population. Again, anti-androgens in an aquatic environment cause problems for male fish.

Are endocrine disruptors – whether they are anti-androgens or anti-oestrogens – really the cause of male fertility problems? There is no doubt about it in the aquatic environment, but despite an explosion of research in this area on humans there is still no definitive data. To say that all of this male reproductive health data is confusing is an understatement. What's particularly hard to comprehend is that effects don't seem to be consistent. Different rates of testicular cancer in nearby countries do not suggest a global contaminant. If rising rates of this cancer are about exposure to oestrogens, why do those countries where phytoestrogens are eaten in the greatest quantities have the lowest rates of testicular cancer? Chemicals with an even weaker oestrogenic effect seem an unlikely cause. Anti-androgens are more likely, although they were introduced after the rise in testicular cancer began. If some of the laboratory research on animal models undertaken by scientists is to be believed, there should be a worldwide epidemic of testicular cancer and infertility – but there is not. If there are effects on male development, why haven't we seen any disturbance in puberty in teenage boys?

This is not to dismiss the clear effects seen in aquatic animals. Nor to applaud the process by which many chemicals have found their way, pretty much untested, on to the market. This is about to change, with knowledge of endocrine-disrupting activity a specific new requirement for licensing. In this sense, *Our Stolen Future* has achieved what *Silent Spring* did in terms of regulation of chemicals, which is entirely proper, although the regulation process, as I have indicated, is unwieldy and will almost certainly have to be modified.

Nevertheless my reading of the huge volume of material on this subject is that changes in diet and lifestyle are much more likely causes of the problems we are seeing with regard to fertility than endocrine disruptors. For instance, in the space of fifty years, the workplace has been transformed: we now largely go to work to sit down and come home to exercise, instead of the other way around. A profession in which you sit all day, such as taxi driver, is associated with poor sperm counts. Paraplegics, fertile before their accidents, may become infertile afterwards, because by constant sitting they are toasting their sperm production factories (their testicles), with their body heat. Less exercise, major changes in diet, increases in smoking and drinking, the deliberate delay in having children, which means couples are more likely to seek help with fertility — all of these will impact on the incidence, or perceived incidence of those conditions for which endocrine disruptors are now being blamed.

As yet there is no definitive evidence of human harm from endocrine disruptors, although this does not mean that there aren't people who have variations of genes which make them more sensitive to inherent or chemically induced oestrogen-related disorders. One must never forget that something which has a very low population risk can still have significant effects. For instance, a one in a million chance of death from something would be regarded by many as no risk, nevertheless would still kill nearly seventy people in Britain.

Many will say that we should be adopting a precautionary principle and safeguarding our children's future by banning chemicals with endocrine-disrupting activity. There is a danger, however, that in doing this you exchange a small theoretical risk for a much bigger real one. Fire retardant chemicals are amongst those with endocrine disrupting activity, yet they save thousands of lives each year. DDT has now been 'unbanned' in some countires because risk of death from malaria was immeasurably greater than from DDT.

This is a polarized debate with vested interests on both sides: at one end are chemical manufacturers desperate not to open the litigation floodgates, but at the other end are researchers for whom endocrine disruptors are a rich seam to mine, with almost limitless sums of money available, particularly from the EU, to study their effects. Every paper in this area finishes with 'more research is needed'. For such a huge research effort to have resulted in so little hard data should tell us something.

One final thought. There has also been a reduction in the male to female sex ratio at birth in Denmark, England, Wales, the USA and Canada. An intriguing paper from Karen Norberg found in a sample of 86,000 births in the US that sons were more likely to be born to women living with or married to their partners before conception. This is an interesting finding, no doubt mediated by hormones and through the same mechanisms that result in greater incidence of boys born to some professions. This social factor could explain why there has been a drop in male births in those countries where an increasing number of births are the result of casual relationships. Hormones respond to social and cultural change as they do to changes in chemicals in the environment.

Hormone Trade Wars

Many people worry about the effect of hormones added to meat. In 1985, the conclusions of the Lamming Committee, a scientific expert working group convened by the EU, that the use of certain growth promoters in animals was safe, was ignored by the EU who banned them. This political risk assessment was to be repeated in 2004 when the EU ignored the advice of its own scientific experts to impose a ban on phthalates. By 1988, the EU had banned the importation of meat from hormone-treated animals – essentially those from the US and Canada – even though yet another committee had come to the same conclusions as the Lamming Committee. It is clear that in both cases, the EU was responding to public concern and placed this above hard evidence.

Some cattle get steroids in their feed, others receive hormones via an implant in the ear. The six hormones involved are three natural types – testosterone, oestrogen and progesterone – and three synthetic ones, trenbolone acetate (synthetic testosterone), zeranol (synthetic oestrogen) and melengesterol acetate. In general, cows are given male hormones and male animals, female ones. Male cattle used to be given a synthetic oestrogen, DES (diethylstilboestrol), which chemically castrated them, enabling them to grow faster. This practice has been banned in both the US and Europe. Veal calves were also being injected with stilbenes, synthetic steroids, directly into shoulder muscle, a practice which left huge local residues. Use of stilbenes has now also been banned in the US and Europe.

There is enormous financial incentive to use hormones, because they increase growth (by around 20 per cent) on less feed – essentially more protein at a cheaper cost. The warnings from the powerful US meat industry that prices would rise if DES were to be banned did not come true; the industry simply moved to alternatives. It is impossible to monitor the levels of the natural hormones, because these vary so much between animals naturally, but meat in the States is regularly spot-checked for levels of the synthetic hormones, which are not permitted to be above a certain tolerance level.

What does this mean for us? Growth hormone is used to increase milk yields, and as many as 30 per cent of American dairy cattle (but not European ones) are treated with the bioengineered version of GH – rbGH. GH is a protein (a chain of amino acids) and does not survive being swallowed. Even if it did, it is too big a molecule to get through the gut. A human infant's guts are different, however, for they are designed for uptake of the big molecules in colostrum, the breast secretion which precedes milk, which will confer the mother's immunity on the baby. Colostrum contains large amounts of insulin-like growth factor (IGF-1), which is the mediator of growth hormone. Athletes take it, believing that it will make them able to absorb IGF-1 just like babies. But I digress. From beefcake back to beef again.

Ultra-sensitive immunoassays are required to detect the tiny levels of hormones present in meat (parts per thousand billion) and this is even before cookong, which destroys most complex molecules. Sex steroids taken orally need to be in relatively high doses or else they don't survive the gut or pass through the liver. This is the reason why hormone levels in the pill or HRT, taken orally, have to be relatively so high. Certainly the levels in meat are infinitesimally small – compared to the sex steroids we eat without a second thought in eggs every day – and tiny compared to our daily intake of phytoestrogens. There is a huge natural variation in testosterone in meat from different animals. Those groups which would be most vulnerable to hormones from meat would be children, in whom the background level of these reproductive hormones is very low, and this includes both sexes during puberty especially.

Cynics would say that the meat trade wars between Europe and the US are less to do with hormones and much more to do with the US producing a cheaper product which would threaten European beef farmers' livelihoods. Certainly there is truth in this, but eating meat boosted by hormones, even if there is no direct evidence of harm, has an undeniable yuck factor. Eating an implant would *not* be good, so they are deliberately put in the animals' ears, which are discarded as waste. What is of real concern is that best practice is not followed by all farmers and what might not be dangerous when practised properly is made so by the activities of a minority.

When the EU ban came into force, opponents argued that controlled use of implants was better than the black market which would follow a complete ban. They have been proved right. A criminal black market in hormone products has developed and their use has been rampant in European feed lots. In Ireland in particular, one substance, clenbuterol which is not a hormone but a type of drug called a beta-agonist – is sold for huge sums to unscrupulous beef farmers. Clenbuterol, which can have potent effects on the cardio-vascular system and airways, does survive in the gut. Growth-promoting cocktails for meat production are sold through the black market and frankly those farmers that buy them have no idea what's in what they're giving to their animals, nor, it seems, do they particularly care. All they know is that they work. So here, it is not hormones but those other additives which are causing problems – partly, it has to be said, because a ban was put in place.

Are hormone residues in meat damaging human health? In Chapter 2 we noted the excess of daughters or sons produced by butchers with changing animal husbandry practices. There have been changes in sex ratio, although these could be accounted for by social factors. Nor are the changes consistent and not all the inhabitants of countries where there has been a change are big meat-eaters.

There was a suggestion that hormones in meat were causing early puberty in Puerto Rico in the 1980s. This led to an investigation by the Centers for Disease Control (CDC). One laboratory found evidence of residues of zeranol (synthetic oestrogen) in the blood of some of the girls who reached puberty early and also in some chicken samples. However, these results could not be verified and testing of beef, poultry and milk samples in 1985 found no hormone residues in any of them. There is still no evidence that, when hormones are used properly, there is any threat to human health. Here we return to the nub of the question. Are they used properly? Eating meat in Europe where hormones are banned is actually no guarantee of non-adulterated meat. While some of us are unhappy about the influence of the big supermarkets, they are generally more rigorous about testing their suppliers' meat than government inspection agencies, because of the risk to reputation if they did not do so.

Hormones will continue to occupy the headlines, with hormones in the environment being the hottest and most contentious hormone issue for some time to come and one that will not be resolved, possibly for decades. In the next chapter, we will turn to something less contentious. The grip that hormones have on our reproductive cycles.

CHAPTER FIVE

HORMONE EXPLOSIONS 3
Hormones as Tyrants

Hormone cycles rule the lives of women during their reproductive years. Fluctuating hormone levels subject us to a monthly roller-coaster of mood and emotion, as well as bleeding, which can be both reassuring and irritating. Periods are the visible signs of a complex hormonal fertility dance, orchestrated from puberty by the brain. Although the menstrual cycles are popularly thought to be inflexible, one following another in a rigorous 28-day march, the reality is actually far more elastic than people imagine and relatively easily perturbed by external influences.

Hormones are blamed for so much during these years. Whatever the problem – mood swings, bloating, infertility, heavy periods – the answer is always 'It's your hormones'. This chapter aims to tell you the truth about these cyclical hormones and also lifts the lid on a cultural hormone phenomenon – the pill.

Hormonally Yours

Let me introduce you – or reintroduce you – to the key players in the wondrous system that runs your reproductive life. From the hypothalamus, we have gonadotrophin releasing hormone, GnRH, and from the anterior pituitary, two key hormones, follicle stimulating hormone (FSH) and luteinising hormone (LH). In an elegantly orchestrated *pas de trois*, the three of them persuade the ovary to produce oestrogens (of several varieties), androgens (ditto) and progesterone. This is how they do it.

Every month, your body gears you up for pregnancy. An egg – not just any old egg, but the pick of the bunch, must be selected for release. Meanwhile, your womb must be prepared for pregnancy, its lining turned from something like a parquet floor into a shag pile carpet, all within the space of a month. This is because if a fertilized egg should appear, it will need that thick and luxurious lining to sink into, settle and implant. If there is no embryo, then the womb lining must be shed, rather than be allowed to continue getting thicker.

There are two parts of your cycle: before and after ovulation. The 'before' section is called the follicular phase, and the 'after' is the luteal phase. Even as you start your period, the level of FSH is beginning to rise. This hormone takes the role of the clerk of the course that waves the flag before horse races. He must get all the runners and riders under starter's orders. Effectively, this is what FSH is doing, for the rising levels have triggered the growth of several wannabe follicles within the ovary.

Every single day of your reproductive life, up to twenty potential follicles are recruited from the store of eggs that you were born with. After a six-month maturing period, just a few will be brought to the finishing line each month by FSH, and only one will win the race to be the dominant follicle that gets to release an egg. Sometimes there is a dead heat, and two eggs are released – which may result in twins.

The chosen follicle becomes exquisitely sensitive to FSH and then to LH. This is enabled by the sudden appearance of a rash of LH receptors. The follicle looks like a ball, containing a small pond of liquid, within which the egg sits. The outer layers of the ball are a steroid-producing factory, pouring out oestrogens, particularly the very potent sort called oestradiol, as well as oestrone. As you will now know from your bluffer's guide (Chapter 1), oestrogens are the final destination steroid, and to make them, you have to make testosterone first. Inside that ultimately girly product, an egg follicle, the male hormone testosterone is being manufactured, before being passed over to different sets of cells within the follicle to be further processed into oestrogens.

These oestrogens escape into the bloodstream. Their effect on the lining of the womb, currently looking thin and pathetic about a week after your period started, is miraculous. Like mustard and cress on a wet flannel, it begins to proliferate and grow. The rising levels of oestrogen in the blood trigger the pituitary to produce a huge whoosh of LH, plus a smaller slosh of FSH. Ovulation will follow within thirty-six hours.

Ovulation predictor kits are over-the-counter mini-laboratories which do the chemical testing necessary to pick up this big increase in LH. You are then supposed to go away and bonk madly. But the kits are not necessarily the key to successful conception. First because, if you are restricting your love-making to just once a month, you will have less chance of getting pregnant, not more. Second, there is nothing that wrecks love-making more effectively than having to do it; and third, just because you have a spike of LH doesn't always mean that you release an egg, as you will see. It's normal not to occasionally. Save your money and buy exotic underwear instead – it's far more likely to be effective.

When the egg is released, the follicle is a bit like a pricked balloon. But LH engineers some reconstructive work and the busted follicle turns into a corpus luteum (yellow body). By now, you are three weeks into your cycle and the corpus luteum is secreting progesterone. It needs to do this for two reasons. First, in order to complete the work on the womb lining that oestrogen has already begun: progesterone will add structure by initiating curious spiral blood vessels, secretory cells and so on, which will ensure the lining is ready for pregnancy. The second task of the corpus luteum is to be the principal supplier of hormones to support pregnancy in its first ninety days.

If you haven't got pregnant by around day 26, the corpus luteum gives up, folding in on itself. There is a sudden drop in oestrogen and progesterone levels. Because progesterone was maintaining the secretions within the womb lining, they suddenly stop too and fluid is sucked from the lining back into the veins. The tissue collapses and the spiral arteries buckle and then rupture, haemorrhaging blood. They are swiftly closed at source (otherwise you would bleed to death) but the blood and the tissue built up so carefully are sloughed off and expelled through the vagina.

Then the whole thing starts all over again. It is downright miraculous – and happening in a body near you, every month.

This cyclical hormonal change also affects the consistency and acidity/alkalinity (the pH) of the cervical mucus. Trying to get through the mucus in the 'after' phase of the cycle is tough for a sperm because, thanks to progesterone, it is not only like swimming in treacle, but highly acidic treacle at that. By contrast, the mucus in the 'before' phase is watery, abundant and clear and the perfect pH for a sperm with an eye to the main chance. The progesterone-only pill exploits this effect, making the cervical mucus so hostile that fertilization is unlikely.

The 'before' part of the cycle is of more variable length than the 'after'. Once ovulation has occurred, it is pretty consistently 14 days to your period – but 12–17 is still normal. Quite a number of cycles – and this is especially the case at the beginning and end of your reproductive life – are anovular. No egg is released. You will still have a period because oestrogen will still have started the growth of the womb lining. When, because there is no egg, its levels fall, menstruation is initiated. Anovular cycles mean that there is no progesterone (because there is no corpus luteum). As it is principally progesterone that initiates period pain (but does not causes it), anovular cycles are painless. There's an explanation of this seeming contradiction later.

The Statistics

The average woman in Britain will have approximately 400 periods in her lifetime. Amongst the Dogon tribe of Mali (who have on average eight babies each), only 110 periods will be experienced, which is just as well since during their menses they are banished to a menstrual hut. There is still much folklore attached to menstruation. Even in Britain, some mothers still tell their daughters not to wash their hair during a period, pursuing a long held and mistaken belief that women are more vulnerable to infection at this time.

An extraordinary American, R. F. Vollman, made menstruation his life's work, compiling a classic volume called simply *The Menstrual Cycle*, which was published in 1977. He based his book on 691 women born between 1875 and 1951, aged from 4 to 63. Age at first period ranged from 9 to 21, with 55 per cent of them aged 13–14. He noted the similarities in menstrual onset between sisters and mothers and noted that the average cycle drops from 35.1 days at 12 to 27.1 by 43. It then rises to 51.9 at age 55.

One of the things admirably shown by his work is the huge variation that is 'normal'. The 'monthlies' are well named, recurring as they do at approximately four-week intervals, yet somewhere along the line it has become an article of faith that a normal cycle is 28 days long. The obsession with 28 is perpetuated with the pill, where women are programmed to bleed at 28-day intervals. Actually, as Vollman showed, only 12.4 per cent of women regularly have cycles of this length, so how has it come to be the gold standard?

In the seventeenth and eighteenth centuries, meddling philosophers liked to translate four weeks as 28 days and very soon numbers were more important than biology. Four times seven for the menstrual cycle and ten times twenty-eight for the duration of pregnancy (forty weeks) became the 'official' length. Thus it is that women, who have come to believe, not surprisingly, that pregnancy is nine months in duration, find when they reach the ninth month, that they still have another month to go. Obstetricians wonder why they do not have a reputation for high-quality research. Given that they are a group of people who, to get the duration of pregnancy, divide forty by four and consistently come up with nine as an answer, it's hardly surprising.

The Moon and You

The length of a woman's cycle is a reflection of her hormones and of her fertility. Those women with cycles of 29.5 days have the highest likelihood of fertile cycles and both short and long cycles are associated with infertility. Is it a coincidence that this happens to be the length of the lunar cycle? For centuries, the moon and menstrual cycles were believed to be linked. When an obsessive Frenchman called Clos actually collected details of the periods of a woman for 289 successive cycles between 1807 and 1834, he claimed, after some complicated sums, that he had proved the link. However, he rather holed his own theory below the waterline by remarking, 'a woman does not always menstruate regularly. Every so often the intervals are shorter or longer.' The one thing that you can guarantee is that a new moon will appear every month – but it is not so with periods.

Since then there have been many more studies, most disproving the theory. But in 1987, an American researcher, Winnifred Cutler, collected cycle details from nearly 1,000 Philadelphia college students, publishing her data in the *Journal of Human Biology*, which showed that the highest density of menstrual onset appeared at the full moon. This means that ovulation would occur at around the time of the new moon, fifteen days before. There was no variation in this with season. A study published around the same time of 826 female volunteers, confirmed these findings; 28 per cent of periods started on the day of the full moon, compared to no more than 12 per cent for any other day of the lunar cycle. In an intriguing adjunct, the levels of melatonin in menstrual blood were recorded in just three of the women and found to peak just before menstruation. Melatonin, the hormone of sleep, is also the slave of the body clock, helping it to coordinate activity in response to changes in day length. Disturbances of melatonin production, for example because of shift work, can play havoc with your cycles, because, in order to maintain your monthly rhythm, the body needs to set its clock each day. It does this with light. If it can't do this, or becomes confused, your rhythms – daily and monthly – become altered.

If all this moon thing seems a bit fanciful and new ageish, perhaps we need to think again. Many animals coordinate their reproductive rhythms, via their hormones, with the moon, and not just those sea creatures like crabs or other marine life dependent on the tides. Flatworms, frogs, hamsters and the monkey species *Ceropithecus* have been shown to do so too. Hormones are the messengers dispatched in response to environmental cues, like day length and phase of the moon, which require appropriate behaviours, like courtship, to be set in motion. Humans are likely to be entrained to some extent by the same environmental cues as other animals, although I doubt, with the night-time light pollution we experience in our own age, that moonlight is still a factor in our lives, as with the Dogon, for whom no reports of moon menstrual phasing have been noted. It has to be said that most scientists are deeply suspicious about the moon having any sort of link with menstruation, thinking the data sets are comparable to those recording itching palms and sprouting hair at the full moon.

But the environment isn't the only thing that can knock our cycles off course.

The Stress Effect

We have talked mainly of LH and FSH, which depend for their production on gonadotrophin releasing hormone (GnRH) being sent from the hypothalamus to the anterior pituitary where messages to increase production of LH and FSH are handed over. GnRH is released not just as one continuous stream, but in little pulsed doses every ninety minutes or so. The effect of stress – in particular, rising levels of the stress hormone cortisol – on the hypothalamus can weaken the strength of the GnRH message, usually through a reduction in the pulsing of GnRH. Many women will notice that during time of stress, their periods – the visible sign of their reproductive cycle and of their fertility – either disappear or become less regular. Certainly extreme stress such as war, burns, sudden bereavement or a serious accident can result in periods disappearing for months. We've already covered the relationship between decreasing levels of body fat and complete loss of periods (a condition called amenorrhoea).

There appears to be a close response relationship between the type and severity of stress and the proportion of individuals whose periods stop. Elevated cortisol levels are also found in women with depression, women athletes and those with anorexia, but not in women with bulimia. These women, including bulimics, all experience problems with their periods. However, you shouldn't think of stress and GnRH purely in terms of levels of cortisol (or of its ultimate master, corticotrophin releasing hormone), or purely in terms of single stressors. Neuroendocrine effects are incredibly complex and multiple, and it might be that seemingly minor psychogenic and metabolic stressors are likely to be more harmful to reproductive function than a single stressor in those that are susceptible. What are these stressors? How long have you got? Commuting, money worries, bullying, uncertain future, long hours, poor relationships – the list goes on and on.

It could be any or none of these, and not just because none of these things might apply to you personally. We each have a very individual response to stress and what's energizing for some brings others down. Our challenges – the metabolic ones (like exercise, nutrition, our level of activity) together with the psychogenic ones (perhaps including performance pressure, negative attitudes, unrealistic expectations, all of which have been specifically associated with missing cycles) – are fed to the brain, which responds by modulating levels of neurotransmitters. The hypothalamus then translates these into altered secretion of its hormones, which in turn affect the pituitary hormones, and through them the endocrine glands. What this means for your periods is nigh on impossible to quantify in relation to a single external force.

There is an equivalent stress effect in men, where the end point is reduction in sperm count. It has always been assumed – on the basis of not very much evidence – that women have a hypothalamus *fragilis* as it's called, while men have a hypothalamus *robustus*. In other words, women are more susceptible to stress. But when US Army researchers actually looked at it, they found that combining a metabolic stressor (fasting) with a psychogenic stressor (a war drill) appeared to suppress GnRH production more profoundly in men than in women.

Stress acting on the hypothalamus can cause many diverse effects, acting through many different hormonal systems – becoming thin for instance, or alternatively, over-eating. Perhaps the bottom line here is that women who miss their periods will pretty soon go to their doctor seeking an explanation. Men have no such visible signs of stress, and if their sperm counts are lower they are unlikely to know unless actively trying to conceive.

It is often said that stress is the reason why couples fail to conceive, and everyone, but everyone, has an example of a couple they know who, having had years of infertility treatment, went away on holiday and conceived – or had two children with IVF and then another quite unexpected one naturally. The implication is that stress must have been the cause all along. It has some influence, but getting pregnant mainly requires two things: time and opportunity for sex.

If a stressed lifestyle means that opportunities for sex are limited to once or twice a month, your chances of pregnancy are immediately diminished. Frequent sex is the cure and going away on holiday is one of the best recipes I know for it. How else do you fill the time between lunch and dinner when it's too hot to lie in the sun?

The longer the period of time that you have been having unprotected sex, the more likely you are to conceive. It is estimated that, with time, a third of the women attending infertility clinics would have got pregnant without treatment. Clearly, if you are thirty-eight, the clock is ticking on, reducing the chances of successful fertility treatment. You're not going to risk it, and hope that you're one of that third who will get there by yourself. You opt for treatment.

Having said this, levels of stress hormones are regulated differently in men and women because oestrogens tend to intensify and prolong the response of the adrenal glands (producers of cortisol). Interestingly, if men are given a short course of oestrogen, they have an increased response to stress. It's possible that testosterone and oestrogen are what determines the body's exact response to stress and perhaps this is why diseases associated with increased amounts of emotional pressure, like post traumatic stress disorder (PTSD), are more common in women than men. Remember, too, that oestrogens have a direct effect on neurons in the brain, not just through the hypothalamus.

The 'Hot Romance' Effect

There have always been anecdotal reports that cycles change during an intense romance (typically that periods intrude early, so ruining your plans for a dirty weekend). Many animals ovulate in response to copulation – cats, for instance, and rabbits. It's called reflex ovulation. For other animals, the mere sight of a male strutting his stuff is enough. It's called the Ram Effect (if you are a sheep). Then there's smell. Young female possums have been shown recently to come into heat simply in response to aromas in male scent trails. So are human menstrual cycles as exposed to outside influence? There are several studies showing that exposure to men has the capacity to shorten menstrual cycles and increase ovulation. In one, researchers showed that women who spent at least two or more nights with men during a forty-day period showed a significantly higher rate of ovulation than those spending one or no nights. This was more the ram effect than the rabbit effect, because ovulation rates were unaffected by the number of times sex took place. There's clearly something about men that literally turns women on. But could there be something about women too?

All Girls Together?

In 1971 a study appeared in journal *Nature* confirming what many women already suspected, that women who share close quarters come to menstruate in synchrony. The author, Martha McClintock, then just twenty-three, based her paper on what she had observed in a dormitory in the exclusive Wellesley College, Massachusetts. Her contemporary and dorm mate was another observant woman, now a US Senator, Hillary Rodham Clinton.

The research came about because when Martha was an under-graduate she had been invited with some other students to a conference about pheromones. Pheromones are airborne chemical signals that are released by an individual into an environment and which affect the physiology or behaviour of other members of the species, without them being consciously detected as odours. The delegates were discussing how they cause female mice to ovulate. In a scene straight out of *Legally Blonde*, Martha tentatively put up her hand and said that the same things happened all the time in humans. When the incredulous scientists said 'where's your proof?', Martha replied that it was what happened in her dormitory.

Her faculty adviser got her to enrol 135 women in her dorm in a study and Martha wrote up the results as her senior thesis. She went on to Harvard and was persuaded by the legendary sociobiologist, E. O. Wilson, who worked on signalling systems in ants, to submit her findings to *Nature*. Nearly thirty years later, Martha, by now Professor of Psychology at the University of Chicago, had another paper published in *Nature* which, she claimed, proved the existence of pheromones.

In the 1971 paper, McClintock considers whether shared light /dark patterns (in other words, room mates sharing the same time for lights out) might be a possible mechanism, with synchrony initiated by melatonin, but rejects this. She noted that synchrony was most noticeable amongst best friends and concludes the paper with 'this indicates that in humans there is some interpersonal biological process which affects the menstrual cycle'.

Although there were mutterings about McClintock's statistical analysis and also about the inclusion of women on the pill, some better designed studies showed much the same thing. That menstrual synchrony was most likely among best friends and women with intensive social contact with each other. However, there were an equal number of other studies showing no such thing and most tellingly, no such correlation was found among lesbian couples.

In 1998, again in *Nature*, McClintock claimed to have proved that pheromones were that 'interpersonal process', which altered the hormones affecting onset of menstruation. In a blinded controlled trial, women were asked to sniff pads taken from the armpits of women in the latter half of their cycle. The sniffers' cycles were accelerated, bringing on their periods earlier than anticipated. Pads taken from women around the time of ovulation had the opposite effect. It was a spectacular paper.

Game, set and match? Well, it's all very curious. This is a

cherished notion which women want to believe, but as most women's periods last five days, and the length between periods is only a month, overlap among a group of women living together is therefore not only possible but highly likely. This is not synchrony, is it? An equally insurmountable problem with this theory is, what would be the purpose of this team menstruation? Not being synchronous with your best mate surely makes having a baby by the best guy around (which is your body's gameplan, if not yours) more rather than less likely. After all, if you are both ovulating, will he sleep with both of you? Not if he values his life he won't. Amongst the cliff-dwelling Dogon, the nearest we have to representatives of early humans, there is no evidence of synchrony, though surely, if it conferred some sort of biological advantage, you'd see it among these women. There is no doubting the existence of human phero-mones, but it's hard to be convinced that menstrual synchrony really exists. If it does, it is a very weak effect.

Bleedin' Awful

In a huge collaborative study on periods, sponsored by the World Health Organization, and involving fourteen different socio-cultural groups across ten countries, including Pakistan, Egypt, the UK and the Philippines, menstruation was associated with youth and sexuality. Overwhelmingly, women do not want to see any changes in their cycles, regarding them as a sign of health, not ill-health. But it does not stop them complaining about 'the curse' – too heavy, too long, too short, too painful, too irregular, too frequent and too awful. Frequently these problems are laid at the door of hormones.

Most periods last between five and six days, with average blood loss of 35 ml. That's seven teaspoonsworth. Heavy periods are defined as blood loss of more than 80 ml but it's what's heavy for you that counts. Women are notoriously bad at estimating blood loss and what's fine for one woman is a catastrophe for another. There are lots of reasons for increased blood loss that have no direct link with hormones – fibroids and endometriosis to name but two. Still most cases of menorrhagia, as it's known in the trade, are unexplained. Prostaglandins – pre-hormones – are usually blamed, along with elevated levels of an enzyme that affects fibrinogen, a party to blood clotting. Despite hormones not being guilty as charged, heavy periods were treated for decades with a synthetic progesterone, norethisterone. It was literally worse than useless. Meanwhile, time and time again, one of the best and most effective treatments was shown to be an anti-fibrinolytic (so an anti- anti-clotting agent) called tranexamic acid. A big clue, you might have thought, yet prescriptions of the synthetic hormone continued. However, using a progestogen-releasing IUD (coil) which slowly releases hormone into the womb cavity does work. Here there is a direct hormonal effect on the lining, which prevents its build-up, and cuts down blood loss that way.

With regard to painful periods, you'd think, given that anovular periods (ones where no progesterone is produced) are painless and that women on the pill don't have painful periods, that hormones – and specifically progesterone – were the villains. Actually that is not the case, at least not directly. Remember, too, that by the time the period actually starts, progesterone levels have been falling for a couple of days. But within all that tissue that is built up during the second half of the cycle are various prostaglandins. Some women develop high concentrations of these, which seem to cause the womb to contract a lot (causing pain). No one knows why this should be so. True, they wouldn't be there if it had not been for progesterone's message to the womb lining to proliferate, but it isn't progesterone causing the pain – honestly.

If painful periods are not quite the fault of hormones, that is not the case with irregular or no periods. As I've outlined earlier, anything that affects the release of GnRH, such as severe stress or anorexia, can cause problems. The commonest endocrine disorder affecting ovulation and causing irregular and disrupted periods is polycystic ovary syndrome (PCOS).

This condition was first described by B. A. Stein and S. E. Leventhal in 1935 (and indeed was once known as Stein–Leventhal syndrome). Women who have PCOS have a triad of symptoms: very irregular periods, obesity and problems associated with too many male hormones, like excess body hair, acne and male-pattern baldness. They also have polycystic ovaries. These are ovaries so packed with follicles, at all stages of development, that they look rather like someone has stuffed them with as many marbles as they could. Although, in fact, ovaries like this are rather common, with around one in five women of reproductive age having them, those with associated symptoms of PCOS are less so, but they still affect around 10 per cent of women.

Problems with another hormone, insulin, add to the misery. Women with PCOS are insulin-resistant – their tissues don't hear the signals from insulin as well as they should. Also, more insulin than normal is secreted, which has a double-jeopardy effect on those androgens. Normally steroids are chaperoned in the bloodstream by steroid hormone binding globulins (SHBG), which mop up all but a small amount of sex steroids. Insulin not only prompts greater production of male hormones by the ovary, but also decreases the number of SHBGs. This means more androgens free to roam about causing trouble. Thus the male hormone effect is enhanced, resulting in greasy skin and acne, hirsutism and even male-pattern baldness.

Not surprisingly, the pituitary becomes thoroughly confused. Its response to this mayhem is to attempt to regulate it with higher than normal levels of LH. But the effect of this is to make ovulation less frequent. One of the consequences of fewer ovulations is a cruel one. Progesterone is released only after ovulation, so women with PCOS who ovulate far fewer times a year than normal are exposed to less of it. Some think that this lack of progesterone predisposes women with PCOS to lay down fat around their middles, rather than other sites in the body. In itself, this fat pattern is associated with Type 2 diabetes.

The consequences on the cycle are very apparent. Great long gaps between periods, or none at all. Meanwhile, obesity further compounds the hormonal problems. In fat cells, circulating male hormones get converted into weak oestrogens. Their effect is to make the womb lining grow and grow, resulting in not just shag pile carpet linings to the womb, but something more akin to a mattress. Because there is no progesterone in anovular cycles, it doesn't get shed as normal. When the woman does eventually have a period and all this lining is lost, her period can be catastrophically heavy.

Infertility is very common although still some women conceive spontaneously, since there are still between two and six ovulatory cycles a year. But inducing ovulation in women with PCOS – who, remember, already have an ovary full to bursting with follicles – is very hazardous, with multiple pregnancy (and we are talking quads and above) a serious risk.

Hairy, fat and infertile. Thanks, or no thanks, to their hormones, these women have been dealt a very poor hand. What used to be a tragedy has now, in the last decade, turned into an endocrine success story. It has been realized that losing weight and taking more exercise in themselves result in an 80 per cent ovulation rate. Combining this with drugs normally given to diabetics increases this further. For those that need ovulation induction, there is now a cunning protocol of gonadotrophins, which are used in carefully stepped doses to just tip the threshold for producing FSH. This allows only a few follicles to be recruited, instead of the many that would have resulted had there been too big a blast of FSH. We'll return to the subject of fertility and infertility anon, but let's now examine the variations in female physiology imposed by variations in hormone levels.

Menstrual Cycle and Disease

The variation in hormones levels over the cycle causes far-reaching effects throughout the body. For instance, hormones can affect the way that women's bodies process drugs. Sometimes women with epilepsy will have a seizure just before or during the first days of their period, something called catamenial epilepsy. This is not just variation in the condition across a cycle as used to be thought, but also a reflection of the fact that many anti-epileptic drugs are metabolized through an enzyme pathway called CYP 3A4. The activity of this system is accelerated by progesterone in the second half of the cycle, so that drugs are cleared more quickly from the body and may be temporarily less effective in preventing fits. Much the same thing happens with the asthma medication methylpredinsolone, which is metabolized differently at different times of the cycle. Many women with asthma may need to alter their medication in line with their cycles. Another example of a drug hormone interaction is the anti-coagulant drug warfarin, which competes for the same blood-binding proteins as oestrogen. This means anti-coagulation may be more marked in the first half of the cycle when oestrogen diminishes warfarin's ability to bind, so freeing more of it to work.

Women report many other conditions which seem to fluctuate across their cycles, particularly autoimmune diseases, which affect far more women than men. For instance, rheumatoid arthritis and MS symptoms both appear to be worse at the beginning of a period. This is because ovarian hormones modulate autoimmune illness. Hormones are clearly not the whole story here, because those women who have specific hormone problems affecting their ovaries don't have a higher than normal incidence of these illnesses. Also, while rheumatoid arthritis and MS tend to get better in hormone-awash pregnancy, lupus (another autoimmune disease) gets worse. What's going on here? Autoimmune diseases occur because the immune system becomes unable to distinguish what is you from what is foreign in you. It then starts attacking you, instead of the foreign invaders it is supposed to deal with. One suggestion – of many – as to why autoimmune diseases are more common in women, is that female sex hormones influence the development of the thymus gland. This is an important site for the production of those bits of the immune system that tell self from non-self.

Whatever the reason for the disparity in autoimmune disease between the sexes, there is definitely a difference between the day-to-day working of men's and women's immune systems. Testosterone dampens the immune system and oestrogen boosts it. Viral infections are less severe in women than in men; parasitic infections are more common in male animals than female ones and so on. Variations in oestrogen across the cycle are likely to be the reason why women report a greater rate of infection of cold sores, for example, just before a period.

Something else that is modulated by hormones is pain. Oestrogen influences the size of the 'field' of nerves activated in response to a painful stimulus. Oestrogen stimulates release of the body's own opioid painkillers. Pain is least noticeable, then, when progesterone as an anaesthetic is at its highest level in the second half of your cycle. This may be an important piece of scheduling knowledge if you are set on having a Brazilian. Does it mean that women are more sensitive to pain than men? No. Whatever our cultural beliefs about tough men, there is no variation between the genders, but a huge individual variation both in response to pain and to pain relief. You see this most dramatically after surgery when patients are able to set levels of pain relief for themselves using what are called patient-controlled analgesia (PCA) pumps. There is a fourfold variation in the 'right' level of pain relief, and there is no correlation with gender, race, age, weight or type of operation.

It's Your Time of the Month, Isn't It?

The most noticeable effect of your menstrual cycle is on mood – which, as a woman, it rather irks me to have to admit. It is true, there is nothing more irritating, or more likely to make you pick up the bread knife and plunge it into the man in your life, than him saying, as you make some perfectly sensible point, 'It's your time of the month, isn't it?' Men have a nasty habit, particularly if they live with you or know you well, of being spot on with this observation. By the way, it is perfectly acceptable for a woman to lie through her teeth when challenged in this way. On interrogation, several men of my acquaintance claimed that their ability to tell whether a woman is hormonal is akin to that of being able to tell whether there is an elephant in the sitting room. I have of course rejected this inform- ation as being prejudiced nonsense. Why? Because I say so.

On a more serious note, pre-menstrual syndrome is a classic model of the way that hormones affect mood and emotion. It is also a fascinating model of fluctuating medical beliefs, swayed by prevailing medical dogma.

Only 10–25 per cent of women between the ages of eighteen and forty-five experience no fluctuations in mood or physical symptoms through their cycle. About two thirds report changing mood and bloating, and of these 10 per cent think this is troublesome enough to consult a doctor. About 3 per cent are severely handicapped by their symptoms for fourteen days a month. Thus there is a con- tinuum from nothing to awful. Also, as you will know, even if PMS isn't something that normally affects you, there are some months when you can be unaccountably ambushed by quite irrational pre- menstrual irritation.

Symptoms occur during the second half of the cycle only, with any one or all of the following: depression, anxiety, rapid mood change or anger, which may also be accompanied by a great range of physical symptoms, including sleepiness or insomnia, bloating, headache, and succumbing to comfort-eating or fatigue. Symptoms tend to increase with age and may start after childbirth or post-natal depression. Nearly half of those with severe PMS have a prior history of depression, and in those with bipolar disorder (manic depression) their condition is exacerbated with their cycle.

Doctors argue about the name for this condition. Pre-menstrual tension (PMT) is out. PMS tends to be used for more moderate symptoms while, post-menstrual dysphoric disorder (PMDD) is favoured by psychiatrists for those severely affected. We'll use PMS here.

Right from the time that the ovarian steroids were isolated, that is to say, in the 1920s and 1930s, PMS was characterized as a condition of either hormone excess or deficiency, with either oestrogen or progesterone or both taking prime responsibility. One of the best-known theories was the low progesterone hypothesis of Greene and Dalton in the 1970s. The fly in the ointment has always been that studies of PMS have consistently failed to identify any difference in progesterone levels between women with PMS and those without it. Thus women with PMS have hormones within the normal range and have no abnormality of reproductive endocrine function. Recently attention has focused on neurosteroids – steroids that are synthe-sized in the brain and have acute effects on some of the brain's chem-ical systems and in particular, the breakdown products of proges-terone.

Let's work through PMS, piece by piece. First of all, removing the womb does not stop PMS whereas removing the ovaries (oopho-rectomy) does. If you have no ovaries, there are no ovarian hormones and no ovulation. Since symptoms appear after ovulation has occurred, in the luteal phase, it suggests that it is something about the hormone cocktail in this part of the cycle that causes PMS.

Symptoms disappear in anovular cycles, and if you banish the cycle, for instance by shutting off GnRH at source with what are called GnRH-agonists (agents chemically similar to GnRH that block its action, and hence also block production of FSH and LH and, because ovulation is shut down, oestrogen and progesterone too), you banish the PMS problem. But significantly, if you then add back progesterone and oestrogen, in the same amounts and regimes, in women who've never had PMS and in those who have, only those who have had it before get it again when you restore ovarian steroids. In other words, women who get PMS seem to be especially sensitive to these hormones.

Progesterone gets a particularly bad press, and this is intensified by what happens when post-menopausal women take combined HRT. During the oestrogen-only phase, they are fine. When they take a progestogen, they get cranky and complain of PMS. Compare levels of oestrogen within groups of women with PMS and those with the highest levels have the most severe symptoms, even though oestrogen alone doesn't provoke symptoms. This suggests that there is some sort of additionality effect with oestrogen *and* progesterone. The sum is more than the parts.

For women with mild PMS, taking the pill, which banishes ovulation, seems to help. But for those with more severe PMS, the pill worsens their condition. No matter how the culprit hormones are presented to the body, naturally or synthetically, they are symptom-provoking in those prone to PMS.

Neurosteroids

Now we come to the brain, certain parts of which are awash with sex steroid receptors. Oestrogen receptors in the brain modulate memory and learning, as well as balance and pain perception. Of greater interest here are the breakdown products of progesterone (pregnenolone and allopregnenolone) which bind to receptors of the GABA system. GABA (which stands for gamma aminobutyric acid) is a neurotransmitter, a brain chemical which facilitates messages across neurons. It acts as an inhibitor. Low levels of GABA plus low levels of serotonin (another neurotransmitter) are associated with violence and aggression. High levels of both produce passive behaviour and a sunny mood. Interestingly, the pharmaceutical drugs that also bind to GABA receptors are tranquillizers and barbiturates. But progesterone's breakdown products are even better at binding to GABA receptors than barbiturates are. So here, in progesterone, you have an on-board, in-house tranquillizing system: progesterone can also be used as an anaesthetic in large quantities. Instead of being calmed, however, women with PMS seem to experience a less sedating effect if given pregnenolone than women without PMS.

Low levels of the neurotransmitter serotonin are associated with depression. Insufficient intake of the amino acid from which the body makes serotonin – tryptophan (found in protein foods like cheese, chicken and beef) – worsens PMS symptoms. There is now a large amount of evidence pointing to a serotonin dysfunction in women with PMS, so that drugs that promote serotonin release and prevent its reuptake improve PMS.

So hormones in the brain, hormones from the ovaries, serotonin – how do they all fit together? Numerous animal studies demonstrate that the serotonin system and ovarian steroids are linked. The evidence is harder to find in humans, but oestrogen given to postmenopausal women is known to increase serotonin. Also women undergoing assisted conception, who experience a decrease in oestrogen, have a simultaneous rise in depression and anxiety, a feature of falling serotonin levels. Thus it's not just the stress of their treatment causing them to feel miserable and low, but a physiological response to lowered oestrogen. Women with PMS become as sensitive to pregnenolone as women without PMS who are being treated with Sselective Serotonin Reuptake Inhibitors (SSRIs) such as Prozac. If serotonin levels are increased, women with PMS are able to experience the sedating effect of pregnenolone that is felt by women who do not suffer from PMS.

This is hard science but there are two things to take away from it. It shows why taking SSRIs like Prozac, normally prescribed for depression, can help what is seen as a hormone problem. Women are rather suspicious of anti-depressants for PMS because they think that it 'relegates' PMS from a hormone problem to one that is in the mind and confected by the mind. A friend of mine with PMS was deeply upset and hurt when she was prescribed SSRIs. 'Don't they believe me?' she kept saying. 'I'm not a depressed neurotic, just pre-menstrual for heaven's sake, this is a hormone problem.' A prescription for an anti-depressant SSRI isn't a value judgement. It's an acknowledgement of the mechanics of PMS. The second thing I hope I've demonstrated – and this is the only time you are going to read this phrase in this book – is that you haven't got a hormone imbalance. Your hormones are balanced just fine – you've just got rather enthusiastic receptors.

One of the noticeable features of PMS is carbohydrate craving – particularly for chocolate. Taking in carbs will certainly up your serotonin – incidentally the biggest serotonin hit is estimated to be from a white bagel and jam. But it's a short-term solution and sets up a vicious cycle as your blood sugar alternately plunges and soars. Low blood-sugar levels also prompt the release of gluco-corticoids, which, as their name suggests, help control glucose. Eating little and often seems to help and choosing foods wisely so that you include complex carbohydrates rather than quick-hit ones may be all you need to do to alleviate your problem. There are a number of books to help you, principally available from the Women's Nutritional Advisory Service.

Stress Again

Before leaving PMS, let me mention stress again. It is always said that stress is a trigger for PMS – certainly its worst aspects always seem to coincide with domestic disaster or travel hell. Actually there isn't a natural variation in stress response with the menstrual cycle, nor is there any difference in stress hormones between women who have PMS and those who don't. However, in women who are affected, there is an increased stress response in the luteal phase. Learning how to manage stress and not let your kids/partner/life wind you up so much is likely to help alleviated the worst symptoms if you have PMS.

The stress response and depression share much in common. In some ways, depression can be understood as an endocrine disease, although it is not often recognized as such. What the stress response does is prepare body and mind for fight or flight. Heart rate goes up, body fuel is mobilized, while anything surplus to immediate requirements (sleep, reproduction, feeding, growth) gets put on hold. There is preferential access to stored memories involving similar experiences, which might help in dealing with the current situation. Behaviour is modified from the normal, cognitively complex exploration of novel circumstances, to well-worn, get-out-of-here-now behaviour. These responses are induced by nor-adrenaline and by cortisol, both produced by the adrenal glands in huge quantity. While short-term stress can be life-saving (and often life-enhancing), chronic stress is almost always bad news, the sufferer experiencing a wide range of symptoms including becoming withdrawn, jumpy, having problems with sleep, losing sex drive or appetite.

Compare this with depression. A person becomes withdrawn, jumpy, has problems with sleep, loses sex drive or appetite. In depression, anxiety is directed at yourself, not at a tiger trying to eat you. The depressed person also has preferential access to memory – but to those memories of past loss and failure. Equally, people with major depression have sustained high levels of cortisol, just as those with chronic stress do, putting them at risk of premature heart disease and diabetes in just the same way as those exposed to constant stress. The realization of the relationship between stress hormones and psychiatric disease opens up a whole new field for diagnosis, treatment and prevention of depression, plus an understanding of the endocrine abnormalities that underlie it.

Contraception – A Brief History

The story of how people have attempted to control a woman's cycle and with it fertility is a fascinating one, and like most of hormone-ology, driven by larger than life people, no doubt driven by their hormones.

Dr Ludgwig Haberlandt was an Austrian doctor who, in 1908, expressed what many doctors felt at the time – that there must be a better method of contraception than the Dutch cap, a simple circle of material which fitted over the cervix, which was all that was available. When in 1916, two German researchers showed that ovulation could be prevented in female animals if they were injected with an extract from the corpus luteum, Haberlandt saw that hormones might be a way of providing safe, temporary, sterilization. In 1919, he transplanted the ovary of a pregnant animal to one that had readily become pregnant before. The rabbit became infertile. He successfully and temporarily sterilized five out of eight rabbits. By 1927 Haberlandt was suggesting that women might be also be temporarily sterilized if they were given extracts of ovaries of pregnant animals. He was vilified in the German press, with one eminent doctor saying that it was a highly immoral act which would permit a few drones of society to indulge in love games – adding for good measure that every scientist knew that there were no such things as hormones of the ovary.

In 1930, the possibility of hormonal contraceptives was raised at the Seventh International Birth Control Conference held in Zurich, but it was all theory because it was still not understood which hor-mones they were actually talking about. But seven years later, there was the first breakthrough with progesterone. Scientists from the University of Pennsylvania tested progesterone, then a fabulously expensive commodity, for its contraceptive effect in rabbits. It worked like a charm, but this research was never taken up. Perhaps this was because, during the war years, almost all endocrine research was directed towards the function of the adrenal glands, so important in shock and battlefield injury. Another important factor at the time was that research was mainly concerned with improving fertility, rather than restricting it.

The Indiana Jones of the Hormone World

Russell Marker was a maverick chemist. He walked out on his Ph.D., choosing not to complete his thesis, then went into hydrocarbons research, where he developed the octane rating system for petrol. This also failed to inspire him and he drifted into yet another field of research. Finally, in 1938, when he was approaching forty, he decide to work on steroids at Pennsylvania State University.

At this time progesterone was available, but the production process was so involved and laborious that it was prohibitively expensive. Marker knew that certain plants contained a substance called saponin, which foams in water, hence their use by primitive peoples as soap. Saponins are also steroids. The one known source of saponins was the plant used to make the drink sarsaparilla, but again this was extremely expensive. Marker read up on botany before going on an expedition to Mexico where he found his steroid source in the wild yam, Dioscorea. He collected two sacks full, and then promptly lost them. He apparently had to bribe a policeman in order to get them back. Once back in his lab, he isolated the yam's saponin, diosgenin. From this, he was able to make testosterone in eight steps, or progesterone in just five. He took his discovery to two different drug companies, who turned him down flat – a move reminiscent, in terms of commercial opportunities missed, of the record company Decca turning down the Beatles.

So Marker withdrew all his savings, resigned his job and moved to Veracruz, Mexico. He harvested ten tons of yams from the jungle and set up a lab in his bedroom to make steroids from them. He offered to sell some progesterone to a Mexican businessman, who offered him $80 a gram, no doubt expecting a few grams at most. Marker then handed him over 3 kg, worth $240,000 at 1943 prices – the equivalent of several million today.

Marker formed a company called Syntex with a German scientist and a Hungarian businessman, finding both his associates from the phone book. There was a dispute over profits and Marker pulled out, taking the secret of a crucial step in the process with him. Syntex eventually managed to work it out, making first testosterone and then finally oestrone from diosgenin. The price of progesterone plummeted to $1 per gram.

By 1949, Marker, surely the Indiana Jones of the hormone world, had retired from research altogether, but his discovery led directly to a synthetic hormone used in 50 per cent of today's contraceptives.

Marker's place at Syntex was taken by a young American chemist called Carl Djerassi, who was recruited to Mexico as director of steroid research. Djerassi and his boss George Rosenkranz discovered a synthetic variant of progesterone, norethisterone, which they were to patent in 1951. Both this product and a later one produced by Searle, norethynodrel, were not, however, marketed as contraceptives – which is what they were – but as products to treat menstrual disturbance.

By the late 1940s, there were perhaps only a dozen people clinically testing contraceptive methods, most in the employ of pharmaceutical companies. The direct impetus to do more came from two extraordinary American women, Margaret Sanger, an American woman's rights activist, and Katherine Dexter McCormick, a science-trained philanthropist.

Margaret Sanger was born in 1883 into an Irish working-class family. She witnessed her mother's slow death, worn out by eighteen pregnancies and eleven live births. Margaret worked as a nurse and midwife in the poorest parts of New York City. What information about contraception there was, was suppressed by the Church and doctors, although the rich and educated could use subterfuge to buy 'French' products (condoms) and 'feminine hygiene products' (spermicides). Sanger defied Church and State, writing a series of articles entitled 'What every girl should know' in her own newspaper, *The Woman Rebel*. She was effectively exiled to Europe in order to avoid the severe criminal penalties she incurred for violating postal obscenity laws. Her case was eventually dismissed and she founded the Planned Parenthood Federation of America. She organized population conferences and mobilized scientists and politicians. H. G. Wells said of her 'When the history of our civilization is written, it will be a biological history and Margaret Sanger will be its heroine.' He was right.

Katherine Dexter McCormick graduated from America's premier science and technology university, Massachusetts Institute of Technology (MIT), in 1904, with a degree in biology. Women students accounted for less than 3 per cent of students. She made many contributions to women's equality, helping to achieve the right to vote for women in 1919. Having inherited a considerable fortune from her husband, she espoused the cause of women in science and when in the 1950s women were still just 3 per cent of students at MIT, she paid for an on-campus residence for women. It helped open the science and engineering professions to them and today MIT has 40 per cent women undergraduates. But it was her funding of the pill, which so significantly advanced women's health and independence, for which she is best remembered.

Sanger was so convinced of the need for simple, reliable birth control that in the 1920s she founded two journals to provide a forum in which scientists could present their research findings. The German doctor Haberlandt had effectively committed professional suicide simply by speaking about contraception, and with his vilification still fresh in their minds scientists were reluctant to work in such a controversial area. In 1951 Sanger was sixty-eight and time was running out, but then she found her scientist, Gregory Pincus. He was an endocrinologist who had fallen foul of the authorities at Harvard, following the publication of a controversial paper on parthenogenesis (virgin birth). He had built a major research organization, the Worcester Foundation, outside Boston, but always had trouble attracting grants. He approached the pharmaceutical company G. D. Searle and persuaded them to go into the hormone business, but their interest was not in contraception.

Sanger visited Pincus and persuaded him of the need for hormonal contraceptives. Equally important, she persuaded her very rich friend, Katherine Dexter McCormick, to bankroll Pincus. Sanger must have been an extraordinarily persuasive woman, for she also managed to convince Searle, who were deeply sceptical that there was any future in this area, to provide the compounds they were developing for use in other areas of medicine, for testing as contraceptives. Without Sanger and the women's movement, there is no doubt that the development of chemical contraception would have been delayed by many years.

The next stage was clinical testing, and Pincus formed a collaboration with John Rock, professor of gynaecology at Harvard. There was a serious problem, however. Progesterone was far more active if given by daily injection, which clearly wasn't a practical option. Given orally, a very large dose was required, which would make it too expensive. Pincus then asked all the pharmaceutical companies to send him synthetic compounds to test, which could be given by mouth without losing their efficacy. Over 200 arrived and he whittled it down to two companies: Searle (with whom he already had a working relationship) and Syntex. Later he worked with Searle alone using their norethynodrel.

Pincus was the pivot between clinic and pharmaceutical company. All of this was carried out in the state of Massachusetts, where birth control was outlawed. Rock's fertility clinic provided the perfect cover for something that was strictly illegal. Their first trial was known as the pee, pee, pee project because of all the urine samples they required women to give for testing (actually PPP stood for Pincus Progesterone Project). The first public presentation of this work by Pincus in 1955 was received with yawns. Concern was raised too about side effects, such as headache.

No trials could be organized in Massachusetts, so the first were carried out amongst medical students in Puerto Rico. They were pretty disastrous, as the students dropped out when they graduated. Subsequent tests on psychotic prisoners weren't helpful either.

In 1956, trials moved back to Rio Piedras, a slum area of Puerto Rico. the pill was considered a technological fix for the burgeoning population problem, then a greater world concern than it is now, and limiting of family size was thought to be a necessary requisite to economic development. Puerto Rico was the perfect testbed. Hormones thus became slaves to a political ideology.

The first trials worked well until the chemists removed 'impurities' from the pill – which turned out to be oestrogen. The consequence was breakthrough bleeding and some pregnancies. Putting oestrogen back solved the problem. Thus the combined oral contraceptive was created.

So how does the pill actually work? By adding oestrogen to your system, the pituitary thinks that it doesn't need to produce FSH, and because this isn't produced there is no recruitment of follicles. If there are no follicles, there is no feedback of oestrogen to initiate a surge of LH which would induce ovulation. Even if there were, the pill is a combined contraceptive containing a progestogen which also acts to stop that whoosh of LH from being produced. No LH surge, no ovulation. No ovulation, no egg. No egg, no pregnancy.

The original dose had, frankly, been a guess. Second-generation pills halved the dose, and then halved it again. Early pills gave as much progestogen a day as is now dispensed in a month. A pill-free interval was created to imitate periods. In effect these are caused by stopping the pill and they are technically hormone-withdrawal bleeds, not periods. There were concerns about side effects then, particularly nausea, and from the start there were worries about breast cancer and thrombosis.

Taking the pill does increase your risk of breast cancer by a very small amount while you use it. But the risk disappears within ten years of having stopped taking it. Since women's risk of breast cancer rises with age, this finding is much more significant for older women than for the younger women who would normally use the pill. The advice would be to consider another contraceptive method from the age of thirty-five. There is no relation between *duration* of use and breast cancer risk. It is thought that the oestrogen element of the pill may promote existing cancer, rather than initiating new ones. Incidence of breast cancer is not the same as deaths from breast cancer. Deaths from breast cancer, in both current and past pill users, are no different from those in non-pill users.

Professor John Guillebaud has translated the most recent epidemiological studies into real numbers. Think of two concert halls each filled with 10,000 women aged forty-five. One lot have taken the pill for varying lengths of time, but stopped when they reached thirty-five (which is very common). The other group have never been pill users. In the never-used group there are ten cases of breast cancer, in the pill user hall, eleven cases.

On the other hand, the pill protects against both ovarian cancer (a 50 per cent reduction after five years which persists for at least ten years after the pill is stopped) and endometrial cancer (protection for about fifteen years after stopping).

There have been many scares about use of the pill. Those concerning deep vein thrombosis perhaps best illustrate the duality of thought and the separation of act and consequence that the pill has created. In 1995, there was a flight from so-called third-generation pills when research revealed that they doubled the risk of deep vein thrombosis (DVT). The consequence was that a lot of women got pregnant. As it happens, DVT is also a well-known complication of pregnancy, caused by blood becoming more sticky. It affects 60 out of every 100,000 pregnant women. But surely it was still safer than being on the pill? Actually no. The chances of getting DVT on those 'high-risk' pills was less than half that of pregnancy at 25 cases per 100,000 women. Women forgot why they were taking the pill. To prevent pregnancy. There was incidentally also a 9 per cent jump in terminations, which, as with any surgical procedure, carry risks associated with anaesthesia – including, of course, DVT.

Survey after survey reveals that from a third to a half of women taking the pill feel unhappy about doing so, mainly because they think that their health is being damaged by hormones or that they are loading their body with unnecessary chemicals. This is hardly surprising for women have been buffeted by scare after scare about hormones – not just the pill but HRT too. I am curious why women continue to take the pill if they are unhappy. There are plenty of other effective contraceptive methods.

There is particular worry that taking hormones for many years will cause infertility. This worry is buttressed by reports from women whose periods do not return when they stop the pill. In fact, work by Professor Howard Jacobs at University College found that amenorrhoea (no periods) was equally common among non-pill-users as in pill users. In some ways this problem is akin to getting on a bus in London, falling asleep and finding yourself in France. The landscape is different because time has passed and you are now somewhere different. Thus it is that problems with your periods, which were not apparent when you started on the pill some five or ten years before, are revealed when you stop it. If you hadn't been taking the pill, with its reassuring withdrawal bleeds, you would have noticed something was amiss much earlier. The difficulty here is that doctors often talk about 'post-pill amenorrhoea' as if this were an actual condition (which it isn't) and use this as an excuse to delay investigation. If this is you, your lack of periods is almost certainly down to some other problem, which should be investigated without delay.

Women who find they have no periods after pill use beat themselves up about it, believing that they have caused their problems and will now not be able to conceive. First, you didn't do this to yourself and second, methods for ovulation induction are now highly successful. As for the pill causing infertility, early studies revealed no difference in fertility for users and non-users, although there was a delay of some three months in conception for pill users having a first baby. However, I suspect that this may be because of widely given advice to 'clear the pill out of your system' before conception. In 2002, a large study of over 12,000 by Farrow showed exactly the opposite of what is believed – that prolonged use (more than five years) was associated with *decreased* risk of delay. The reason for waiting to conceive after coming off the pill, incidentally, is because one of the effects of the pill is to reduce the level of folic acid and other vitamins in the body. Folates are important in preventing the type of handicaps called neural tube defects, which include spina bifida.

Should the side effects put you off? You need to remind yourself why you are taking the pill and ask yourself, what would happen if you fell pregnant. What impact would a baby have on your life and how would you cope? Now compare that with the known risks as you perceive them. We all look at risk through different glasses and for some breast cancer is a major fear despite the risk being a very small one. To me, the concerns about DVT are more puzzling, because if you get pregnant you immediately put yourself naturally, as we have seen, at much greater risk of this complication. It's a decision that you have to take for yourself, but the bottom line is how important avoiding pregnancy is to you.

One further point, which illustrates a recurring theme throughout this book, is about being uniquely hormoned. If you have side effects when you take the pill – breakthrough bleeding, greasy skin, mood change, breast soreness are the commonest – swap to another brand. Women are very individual and even the tiniest change in the hormones you receive can make a difference to you. A small number of women, however, will never 'get on' with the pill and if this is you, just jump ship to an IUD.

The other point about being uniquely hormoned is that missing a pill matters more to some women than others – especially the sort, I suspect, who later says that their husband only had to unzip his trousers for her to get pregnant. What you are doing during the pill-free interval is allowing the ovary to escape from its imposed hormonal straitjacket. In a study from the Margaret Pyke Centre, 23 per cent of women were, by the end of their pill-free period, developing follicles again and two of those women were within two days of ovulation. Had they missed taking the first couple of pills in the new packet and had sex, they would have probably have got pregnant. Lengthening the pill-free interval is a sure way to decrease protection, and in some, a recipe for pregnancy. Beware in particular of missing pills early in the packet.

Despite all the scares, 200 million women are estimated to have taken the pill, which is probably the best-researched pharmaceutical product in the world. It was hailed as giving freedom for women, but fifty years after its introduction one wonders whether the price of freedom has been too high, for there is now an expectation by men that women will control fertility and in some senses, this hormone product for women has been more liberating for men. Some will say that extra breast cancer cases are too high a price to pay for the pill, forgetting that pregnancy leads to birth, something which is still fatal for many women, particularly in those countries without easy access to medical care. There are also those who would say that the pill has caused an explosion in promiscuity and taken innocence from young women. Have you met any young women en masse lately? If I were an adolescent boy, I would be very afraid.

the pill has always been closely entangled with sexual politics. Control of reproduction, and hence of sexuality, has always been a matter for suspicion, if not outright hostility, particularly from those quarters where control has been usurped. It seems to me that news of side effects of the pill, many of which were scares but some of which were accurate (especially those concerning smoking and cardiovascular effects), have always been seized upon with special glee, as if women deserve everything they get for trying to subvert nature. The subverting nature argument is a curious one. Polio vaccinations subvert nature, so do kidney transplants, but we don't view them as such – but then neither have anything to do with sex as the pill does. That is its great threat.

Infertilty

We have talked of fertility and the pill and covered one of the common, hormonally induced causes of infertility, PCOS. Another hormonal cause of infertility is a luteal phase defect (LPD). Basically the womb lining isn't in the right place at the right time. To get that wonderful shag-pile effect, progesterone is required. In LPD, either because the follicle isn't good, or because the corpus luteum packs up before it should, the womb lining hasn't had the progesterone needed to do its thing, so no implantation will take place. Extra progesterone or other hormones are used as treatment.

Infertility and its treatment is a complex and growing field, which is too large to cover here, but I did want to draw your attention to one fact. Whatever the cause of infertility – and there are many, including straight plumbing problems like blocked tubes – hormones are almost certain to be used in treatment. In fact, without the manufacture of hormone-based drugs, IVF would not be possible, nor would many of the very successful treatments now available.

Let me briefly introduce some of the main hormone treatments used in infertility treatment. Clomiphene (Clomid) is a first-line treatment for ovulation induction – in other words, something that your GP might prescribe. It's an anti-oestrogen which fools the pituitary into thinking that more FSH is needed, which may be enough to kick-start ovulation. You should not take it for more than six months – for no other reason than if you aren't pregnant by this time, you and your partner need a more thorough assessment of your needs and there is no point in delaying it.

Human menopausal gonadotrophin (Pergonal, Humegon) is used in a clinic setting, after more detailed investigations, and is a mixture of two hormones, FSH and LH. Injections are given daily, so that the ovaries begin developing follicles. These are followed 7–12 days later by an injection of human chorionic gonadotrophin (the hormone of pregnancy), which tells the ovaries to release the eggs that have been developed. More than 75 per cent of women will ovulate with this regime of drugs.

Initially, these drugs were produced using millions of gallons of human urine. Yet, no matter how refined the processing, the drugs still contained impurities. But in the mid-1980s, bioengineering became possible, and in 1997, the two principal companies in this market, Serono and Organon, announced recombinant DNA versions in which bioengineered cells produce the hormone, rather than nuns. Hormones produced in this way combine very high purity and very specific biological activity. They have fewer side effects and are more effective. Recombinant technology is now the main method of manufacturing hormones.

This chapter has been about the 'juicy' hormonal years, those from roughly from thirteen to fifty. What happens when this regular cycle disappears and hormones crash is the subject of our next chapter.

CHAPTER SIX

HORMONE CRASHES

We have seen how hormones rule women's lives during their reproductive years. Although some may complain about their periods, they would still rather have them than not. That monthly bleed is a reassuring constant both of health and of womanhood.

But from the age of about forty-five, it becomes clear that your periods are not as they were. The pattern changes, losing that familiarity of what has become normal for you. Shorter, longer, heavier, lighter, every twenty-three days or at forty-day intervals, there is certainty no longer. Your world is changing and your body is in hormonal revolt, with your ovaries apparently deaf to the increasing volume of internal hormonal messages arriving on their doorstep, from the pituitary gland in the brain. Your reproductive hormones are about to crash, to less than 10 per cent of their former values. They are also about to become villains.

The effects of repeated cycles and of the body's exposure to sex steroids, so welcome at one time, are now increasing susceptibility to breast, ovarian and endometrial cancer. Without oestrogen to bathe the tissues, skin thins, fat redistributes itself, hair dulls, cognition becomes woolly, sex less important. This is the menopause. Although their hormones drop less precipitously, men too experience a steady decline of their hormones with age. The effect of these hormone crashes is momentous. So too is the decision whether to replace what has been lost and what with, and this decision has had a major cultural impact on society.

The Menopause

The menopause has been deemed a kind of physiological 'terrorism', but to blame hormones in this instance would simply be shooting the messenger. The word itself comes from two words of Ancient Greek, *menos* (a month) and *pausos* (an ending), hence our word *menopause*, which strictly means the end of the monthly or menstrual cycles.

By the age of twenty weeks, a female fetus already has between six and seven million eggs, which given that we are only likely to have 450 cycles in our lifetime, is monumental over-provision. A process of reduction begins soon afterwards and by birth we have between one and two million. When we hit puberty we have only 400,000 and by the time we get to menopause, that's it, we have no more. But you're right, the maths doesn't add up. It is estimated that 99.998 per cent of our eggs go to waste, having been rejected, zapped, shrunk or left by the wayside, with just 450 or so eggs being selected as stars, destined for ovulation.

The average age of menopause in Britain is fifty-one, yet there is evidence that once upon a time it occurred *earlier*, at around forty or so. It still does so in parts of the developing world, and this probably reflects, since eggs are made in fetal life, the better nutrition in pregnancy enjoyed in the developed world. Nevertheless the age of menopause, unlike the age at onset of periods, has been reasonably constant over the last century. This may alter, since obesity – which is rising – results in a slightly later menopause. Regular smoking can also bring it forward by two years.

The ovary is a bit like a giant egg-timer, set for roughly fifty years. It doesn't run at a constant rate, but speeds up dramatically after the age of thirty-seven, with egg numbers halving every three years, instead of every seven years before this age. If there weren't this late rush, it has been estimated that our eggs would last until the age of seventy. The fall in the number of eggs can also speed up dramatically if eggs are destroyed for any reason, through chemo-therapy for cancer, or autoimmune disease, for instance. This would then result in premature ovarian failure and menopause before the age of forty.

Although taking the contraceptive pill suppresses ovulation, unfortunately that doesn't mean that you can eke out your egg store and have a later menopause. Five years' worth of cycles is just sixty or so eggs, trivial in comparison to the thousands being lost each month. Anyway, if this were true, women who had many pregnancies (and so fewer ovulations) would have a later menopause too – but they don't. Incidentally, if you start periods earlier, it doesn't mean that you finish earlier, having got through your store ahead of time. In fact, if anything it's the reverse: women who start earlier simply seem to have more on their egg-timer clock than those who start late.

If you could count how many eggs were left in the ovaries, you would have a good idea of when menopause was likely to occur – an important piece of information, perhaps, for career women counting on being fertile later in life. Two researchers from Scotland claimed to have cracked this in June 2004 with a new test which used ultrasound scanning of ovarian volume in combination with a mathematical formula. 'Tests that give a deadline for childbirth' in the *Daily Mail* was typical of headlines at the time. In fact, it had never been tested on women, so was a little premature. Menstrual diaries are probably more accurate. When the range between shortest and longest cycles reaches at least forty-three days, you probably have no more than twenty cycles left on the clock and menopause will occur in one to two years. Menstrual cycles not only become more irregular, but are more likely to be anovulatory ones, in which no egg is released at all.

'Menopause' means the end of menstruation, which is a single event. The word 'climacteric' more accurately describes the changes of mid-life, which spans the ages of forty to sixty.

Every month, during the reproductive years, about twenty

follicles compete to be 'the one'. The follicle is a nursing unit. The cells that tenderly enclose the egg, which sits in a puddle of fluid, are actually called nurse cells. They secrete steroid hormones, such as oestrogen and progesterone, into the puddle. Nurse cells and eggs are entirely interdependent – without one, there is no need for the other. As the eggs are killed off, so are the nurse cells. Equally, as you get older, the pituitary gland begins to rev up the production of FSH, perhaps because there is less 'noise' from returning messages provided by oestrogen and progesterone. It might also be that a rising level of FSH is simply a function of chronological age, the first step in reproductive ageing, rather than a consequence of it. Whatever the truth here, the pituitary sends out more and more FSH in an effort to get things back on track, but to no avail. So much FSH is being pumped out, that huge quantities get excreted into the urine. Once FSH gets to a certain level, the writing is on the wall. Menopause will follow as night follows day – and in fact, bloodstream FSH levels are the basis of tests for the menopause.

One woman's hormones, however, can be another's salvation. Because the urine of post-menopausal women contains so much follicle stimulating hormone, it is one of the best sources of the hormone for the induction of ovulation prior to IVF treatment. Thus it was that the urine of nuns living in convents close to the Vatican was collected by pharmaceutical companies. A small donation was made to the nuns for their services and this pee fee went to the very same Catholic Church which condemned the fertility treatments. The demand for FSH was so great that the companies extended urine collection to convents in Eastern Europe. When genetically engineered FSH became available, the demand for menopausal urine from nuns slumped. However, urine-sourced FSH is still available and is considerably cheaper than the recombinant variety. Pharmaceutical companies are cagey about where they collect their urine, but much of it is thought to be from South American women and not even nuns either.

So programmed egg-death destroys the nurse cells, source of the hormones that will help each one achieve its destiny of being the egg that is not only released, but gets to be fertilized and implanted too, thus forming new life. One cancels out the other. If that's the 'how' of menopause, with hormones playing a key role, the 'why' is more tricky. Risks associated with pregnancy, such as life-threatening haemorrhage, increase with age (or more accurately, with the number of previous pregnancies). More importantly, by forty, your eggs, with you since birth, are beginning to show their age just as you are. This means a far greater likelihood of chromo-somally abnormal eggs – it's one of the reasons why older women have higher numbers of miscarriages because even more embryos than normal fail the criteria for implantation imposed by the womb lining. If it weren't for menopause, many more abnormal babies would be born.

In a trade-off between the things that make for a healthy and easy old age and efficient reproduction, there is no contest. Begetting more of us is what we are engineered to do. Everything is geared towards having babies, and frankly, if we die after with our last period, having produced babies that we keep alive until puberty, when they can also begin reproducing themselves, our genes can congratulate themselves on a job well done. Having moist vaginas so we can go on enjoying love-making until our dying day has never been part of the plan. Thus the fact that we experience menopause at all is a consequence of women living longer than allowed in the original grand scheme of human beings. There are some scientists who believe that women are geared to live for an infertile decade after menopause, shepherding their last child through its crucial first ten years while dispensing pearls of wisdom to younger women. I'm not convinced, are you?

So now we have tens of millions of fifty-plus women, with the varied ailments of menopause, from hot flushes ('flashes' if you're an American), sweating and palpitations to insomnia and dry skin. Although some oestrogen is still produced, it is not oestradiol, which is one of the most potent forms, but oestrone, a much weaker oestrogen. And it no longer comes from the ovaries but, of all things, from fat and muscle.

Fat cells contain an enzyme called aromatase, which changes the weak androgens produced by the adrenal glands into oestrone. This is the reason why it is better to be fat than thin at the menopause.

The more oestrone you can get, the less severe your menopausal symptoms. It's also why exercise is so crucial to well-being post-menopause because it too stimulates conversion of androgens into oestrone. One of the ways to self-medicate, therefore, is to indulge in vigorous exercise.

Oestrogen has many hundreds of actions throughout the body and at each site where it's active there are oestrogen receptors, which hook in passing oestrogen and set it to work. There are oestrogen receptors throughout the brain and without it the hippocampus (the site of memory formation) functions less well, making us more forgetful. Certainly women complain of that amnesia moment, forgetting what you are talking about in the middle of a sentence. It is also claimed that cognitive function is affected, with conceptual thinking in particular becoming more difficult post-menopausally. Then there are the well-documented emotional swings that are a feature of mid-life for some – but not all – women, including anxiety, irritability, tearfulness and depression.

Depression is a major complaint of the post-menopausal years but I'm reluctant to lay too much of this at oestrogen's door. Life is about more than hormones and there are many other drivers of depression that coincidentally occur in mid-life: the death or serious illness of a parent, retirement, or your children clearing off and leaving you alone with a man you've hardly spoken to in twenty years, for example.

One of the most noticeable effects of the menopause is on skin, which thins throughout the body, both the bits you can see (more wrinkles) and the bits you can't. The wall of the bladder and the vagina become thin and the vagina tends to dryness, with what secretions it has becoming less acidic, meaning that infections in both vagina and bladder are less easily rebutted.

The idea, however, that the vagina is a permanent desert zone after menopause, with older women incapable of lubrication unless blessed with the contents of a tube of K-Y jelly is simply wrong. Sure, dryness can be a problem and yes, arousal takes longer, but older women (look away now if you are a nervous twenty-five-year-old), once aroused, can lubricate with the best of them. Although female sex steroids are hugely important to sexuality, they are not what drives desire. True, in many animals it is the female sex steroid hormones which limit mating to the period of ovulation. In primates and humans, it is the hormone primarily seen as the architect of male desire and libido, testosterone, that is responsible for women's sexual desires. Oestrogens enable sex, testosterone makes us want it.

In women who have their ovaries removed, libido may disappear altogether – not because of the lack of oestrogen, but through lack of testosterone. It took a very long time for gynaecologists to realize that this was the case. Male hormones remain in our bodies after oestrogen so catastrophically takes flight. The inner cortex of the ovaries continues some sex steroid production, but it is of the male hormones, testosterone and androstenedione. The adrenal glands also continue to produce androgens as they did before the menopause.

To go back to oestrogen, one of the most noticeable effects of lower levels are hot flushes. They are a bit of an enigma and their exact mechanism remains unknown. Apparent surges of heat occur across the whole surface of the body, although women mostly only notice it on their upper half and face. The brain, thinking it's hot, sends signals to the peripheral blood vessels in the skin, telling them to dilate, which allows excess heat to be lost through radiation. Actually, more often than not, it's not hot at all but the brain has been tricked by the strange behaviour of the body's thermostat. It lies very close to the hypothalamus which is the source of gonadotrophic hormones.

It's the long-term effects of oestrogen loss that have been the driver for the hormone wars of the last three decades. Cardiovascular disease (not, please note, breast cancer) is the single most important cause of mortality in post-menopausal women. Arteries are more rigid after the menopause, clotting factors change, cholesterol increases – all risk factors for heart disease. Prior to the menopause, women's risk is lower than that of men, but climbs steadily thereafter. The steadiness of this rise, which starts before the menopause, is interesting because if loss of sex steroids were the only key factors, given a 90 per cent fall, surely the increase in coronary heart disease (CHD) would show a steep sudden rise at menopause? Nevertheless, it is the increase in CHD in older women and the possibility of preventing it that has been one of the principal factors in recent thinking on hormone replacement therapy, of which more in a moment.

Another major consequence of oestrogen loss is in bone density. Oestrogen facilitates full utilization of all the panoply of hormones, including calcitonin and parathyroid, vitamin (D) and minerals (calcium) (Vitamin D, calcium) that are all essential to bone health. Oestrogen also affects the balance between the two opposing camps of cells in bones – the builders and the removers – by favouring the builders and adding oomph to their activity. After menopause, without its influence, the activities of bone-removing cells become greater than those of the building ones, resulting in net loss of bone mass. The condition of thin, fragile bones that are susceptible to fracture is known as osteoporosis, and it is responsible for over 200,000 fractures each year in the UK, as well as great pain and disability. The most common fractures are in the hip, wrists and spine. About a third of women with hip fractures will die within a year, not from the fracture itself, but from the deadly consequences of immobility, such as infection and embolism, that it causes. Those who have osteoporosis typically lose height as their bones crumble, developing a typical 'dowager's hump'. Osteoporosis is partly inherited and is also influenced by lifestyle factors such as smoking, poor diet and lack of exercise. Nor is this just seen at menopause. One of the severest consequences of the disturbance of reproductive hormones seen in anorexic women, ballet dancers and over-exercising athletes is bone loss.

For many years, oestrogen (supplied via HRT) was not just the gold standard treatment for osteoporosis, it was the only treatment. It is only relatively recently that new drugs such as the biphosphonates have become available for treatment of brittle bones. Men (who suffer from osteoporosis to a much lesser degree) are given testosterone – which has an effect on their bone mass only because it is converted by their bodies into oestrogen.

Osteoporosis is a major public health problem, costing the NHS over £1.7 billion annually. Yet it is largely invisible, ignored by the media and public alike because it principally affects old women and causes disabilities we would rather ignore because society regards them as conditions of ageing, rather than as a disease process.

Oestrogen is also a promoter of other hormones, working hand in glove with growth hormone, for instance, to enhance its production. Certainly blood levels of growth hormone drop like a stone at menopause and are restored somewhat with HRT. Might it be that the rising incidence of heart disease after menopause in women is not the direct result of oestrogen loss, but instead something to do with growth hormone? It is now known that the heart is riddled with receptors for IGF-1, the mediator of growth hormone and that low levels of IGF-1 are associated with some types of heart disease in the elderly. It is certainly an avenue for future research.

Hormone Replacement

So there you are. A catastrophic loss of hormones in mid-life. Replacement has to be the answer – or at least, that's what seemed glaringly obvious at the time of Brown-Séquard. Augusta Brown was a Parisian midwife in the early twentieth century and inspired by *La Méthode Séquardienne*, she prepared extracts of guinea pig ovaries, which she injected into older women. She claimed success but since she used water rather than alcohol to prepare her potions, there would have been little, if any, oestrogens in them. But she was possibly the first person to try hormone replacement therapy for women.

Those women who were understandably squeamish about the ferocious hypodermics of the time were urged to eat fresh raw pig or cow ovaries, thinly sliced in sandwiches. There were also many varieties of tablet and sugar-coated pastilles, which were claimed to contain ovarian 'juices'. Although we now know that these would have had no effect, at the time they were hugely popular.

When hormones were first isolated and synthesized, they were drugs looking for diseases to treat. Some illnesses caused by deficiency – diabetes or hypothyroidism – were obvious candidates but sex hormones had less of an obvious market. It is not clear when menopause moved from being a natural part of ageing to being considered a disease of hormone deficiency. Certainly prior to the Second World War there were those, including the renowned endocrinologist Fuller Albright, Professor of Medicine at Harvard, who were beginning to label the menopause as a deficiency syndrome. When, in 1939, Ayerst developed a process of extracting oestrogens from mares' urine, the 'indications' were very modest – relief of menopausal symptoms, principally for those women who had had their ovaries surgically removed. Ayerst marketed Premarin, the very first oestrogen replacement therapy, in Canada in 1941; in 1942 it was approved for use in the United States. Premarin tablets were first available in the UK in March 1956, when they were supplied by Imperial Chemical (Pharmaceuticals) Ltd, and were pills designed for a very specific condition. What the pharmaceutical companies really needed, however, was a much wider 'ill' to treat, if a drug was to be really successful.

Help was at hand. In 1966 a New York gynaecologist and oestrogen cheerleader called Robert Wilson wrote a bestselling book called *Feminine Forever,* in which he likened menopause to ovarian castration. Wilson, who was partly bankrolled by the manufacturers of Premarin, Wyeth-Ayerst, was a strange character with – judging from his prose – an apparently morbid fear of old women. He claims in the book that he could recognize a woman who has had HRT by the 'outward signs of age-defying youthfulness', which are:

a straight-backed posture, supple breast contours, taut smooth skin on face and neck, firm muscles and that particular vigour and grace typical of a healthy female. At 50, such women still look attractive in tennis shorts or sleeveless dresses.

This is how he describes those women not on HRT:

I have seen untreated women who had shrivelled into caricatures of their former selves. Some had lost as much as six inches of height by the pathological changes caused by lack of oestrogen.

No wonder women wanted oestrogen. Within a year, the book had sold 100,000 copies. The resulting enthusiasm for oestrogen replacement meant that sales quadrupled between 1963 and 1973. Half the post-menopausal women in the States were using HRT – and who can wonder, with their shrivelled desiccated future laid out so helpfully before them by Dr Wilson and his acolytes who likened menopause to living decay? Menopause was not a lifechange: it was a disease that required treatment.

Instead of simply being prescribed for symptoms such as hot flushes, HRT gradually became touted as a cure for everything from heart problems to ageing skin and, regrettably, for problems that were mostly not much to do with medicine but about relationships grown stale with age and familiarity – such as lack of a fulfilling sex life. Then came the first reports of endometrial cancer.

In 1975, the *New England Journal of Medicine* published two studies documenting a strong association between cancer of the lining of the womb (the endometrium) and oestrogen therapy. Progestogen (a synthetic form of progesterone) was then added to the monthly oestrogen regimes to protect against the thickening effect (hyperplasia) caused by oestrogen, which can lead to cancer. Oestrogen alone is associated with a 7–15 per cent risk of hyperplasia, which is reduced to 5 per cent when progestogen is added each month (this is called opposed therapy). The risk reduces to zero if progestogen is taken for 12–13 days per cycle. Thereafter, unopposed therapy (oestrogen only) was given only to women who had had a hysterectomy.

Feminism didn't always know what to think of HRT. The right to remain juicy, espoused for a while, quickly became tempered by concern over the use of steroid hormones and the way in which menopause was being medicalized as a disease. Meanwhile, during the 1980s, HRT continued to gather popularity and women continued to demand it, despite a plethora of studies which were indicating increased risks of breast cancer with long-term use.

HRT is now worth about £2 billion a year worldwide. That, plus the wide range of products competing for market share, ensures that it is heavily marketed. But for feminism to deride all those who opt for HRT as victims of a marketing or medical conspiracy – a view typically espoused in Sandra Coney's book *The Menopause Industry: How the Medical Establishment Exploits Women* or as gullible fools in search of lost youth, one of the views taken by Germaine Greer in her book *The Change* – makes a mockery of sisterhood. Women whose lives are made a misery by night sweats, insomnia and hot flushes want something that enables them to live a normal life again, thank you very much, without being told that they are patsies in an androcentric universe. The media, too, has a particularly ambivalent attitude to HRT, with the more misogynistic papers, such as the *Daily Mail*, seemingly seizing on every new study of adverse effects with glee. For surely this is all women's fault for wanting to have it all? No, actually.

Some women just want to sleep through the night without drenching the bed in sweat or living their life as an additional radiator in the house.

Another factor which heavily influences our view of HRT – and indeed of many things – is fear of cancer, or rather fear of one cancer. Breast cancer occupies the highest rung of our fear ladder, because we perceive it to affect femininity during those years when sexual attraction is still important to us. There are many breast cancer charities, all competing for the same pool of money and some among them deliberately exploit women's natural fear of breast cancer. When challenged, they will claim that the end justifies the means – for how are they to raise funds for research otherwise? What they mean, of course, is how are they, rather than their competitors, going to raise funds? Thus breast cancer has been assiduously promoted as a killer that affects one in ten. Of course breast cancer can kill, but four out of five women diagnosed now survive in good health. The news is not so good for colon cancer, against which HRT has a definite preventive effect, but in the game of life, breast trumps bowel every time. Meanwhile osteoporosis, the Cinderella disease hidden behind closed doors, causes chronic disability for the remainder of life and, as I have indicated, kills too. But this disease does not generally appear on the radar because just as teenagers cannot perceive the dangers of smoking twenty years on, neither can fifty-year-old women perceive the dangers of osteoporosis twenty years on. Our HRT riskometer is driven not by the totality of risk, but seemingly by that of breast cancer alone.

The irony is that those who fear breast cancer most are those least likely to be affected themselves. There is indeed a one in ten *life-time* risk of breast cancer, but the chances of a twenty-five year old developing it are vanishingly small. The association of breast cancer with youth, through campaigns which feature young women celebrities, has led those women most at risk – the over-fifties – to assume that it is a young woman's disease. It is not. Age is the single biggest risk factor for breast cancer. Meanwhile, the greatest health risk to older women – coronary heart disease – is also largely ignored.

However, the risks of CHD are not lost on the medical profession. The majority of HRT studies in the 1980s showed a reduced risk of coronary heart disease in users of HRT compared to non-users. Certainly oestrogen has well-documented beneficial effects on the vascular system, but even so there was surprise when some studies suggested an extraordinary drop of 50 per cent. Suddenly HRT became *the* preventive cardio-protective drug. Such extravagant figures should have rung warning bells. The pharmaceutical companies, however, sensing at last the nirvana of a pill for all, instead of a pill for the few, poured money into the marketing of this new wonder drug. But one of the problems of many of these studies was that they compared women who had *chosen* to take HRT. On the whole, they were better educated women, who exercised more, had lower blood pressure and who were more likely to engage in preventive health measures. In other words, like was not being compared to like. Not all was hyperbole, however. There were many more sober studies from a wide range of independent sources showing benefit, which propelled doctors towards recommending HRT. The 20:20 vision afforded by hindsight allows one to say that doctors should have known that they were prescribing something with long-term dangers. But at the time, available evidence showed benefits in terms of cardio protection, which skewed thinking on HRT dramatically.

Opinion was still fiercely divided about HRT. On the one side were the enthusiasts, largely gynaecologists, who called it the greatest preventive drug ever developed, and on the other were those like Germaine Greer, whose piercing analysis of the 'menopause industry' – *The Change* – was published in 1991, who felt sure that menopause was not a disease and that many of the medical theories and treatments were contradictory, excessive and at times dangerous. There were also those in the middle who considered

HRT invaluable, in the short term, to treat women with unbearable menopausal symptoms, but who had no truck with the extremists of either persuasion.

The first suggestion that HRT might not be cardio-protective came in 1998 from the so-called HERS study *(Heart and Estrogen/progestin Replacement Study)*. It showed that HRT did not prevent further heart problems in those women who already had heart disease. This made the idea of protection from heart disease for those who had not yet developed it a less tenable proposition. Since heart protection was now a major part of the equation that made doctors recommend HRT, once this benefit fell away, it suddenly made much less sense as a preventive medicine.

The Women's Health Initiative (WHI) study was a randomized, double-blind, placebo-controlled study that was conceived and carried out in the US in the 1990s. It reported in 2002. It was designed to test the efficacy of HRT on coronary heart disease and had two groups: one of oestrogen-only (5,310 women) and the other of a combined preparation (8,506 women). Women in Britain tend to be prescribed HRT in their forties and fifties, but the average age of the women in the study was sixty-three. The first group was followed up for 6.8 years and the second for 5.2 years. Both were stopped early, the oestrogen-only group because there was an increased risk of stroke and no evidence of benefit for CHD, and the combined group because of the risk of breast cancer exceeding the safety threshold set for the study in advance.

The study found, as expected, an increased risk of breast cancer with the combined preparation but a decreased one with oestrogen only (which was a very considerable surprise and completely counter-intuitive). It found reduced risks of colorectal cancer and fractures with combined use, and increased risk of colorectal cancer, stroke and blood clots with oestrogen only. Neither preparation had a beneficial effect in coronary heart disease; in fact, it seemed the reverse was true.

The headline findings were, to any woman taking HRT,

horrifying – '26 per cent increase in breast cancer, a doubling of clots, strokes increased by a massive 41 per cent, heart attacks by 29 per cent'. In the UK, it was estimated that over 350,000 women stopped taking HRT. I'm astonished it was so few.

As ever, the figures weren't quite what they seemed. Professor David Purdie, an expert on HRT, was challenged by John Humphrys on the BBC Radio 4 *Today* programme on these apparently enormously increased risks. 'I call it the Judas factor,' said Purdie. Intrigued, Humphrys asked what he meant. 'Jesus was betrayed by 8 per cent of his disciples.' 'But surely, there was only one – Judas,' protested Humphrys. 'Precisely my point,' said Purdie. 'Judas was alone among the twelve but he was 8.3 per cent of them. We can easily be misled by the used of percentage values – especially when the numbers are small. That's why you should always insist on absolute values for do you not deserve the absolute truth, not a percentage of it?'

Now let's look again at that HRT study but in real numbers (these were released at the time by the Committee on Safety of Medicines). Of every 1,000 women aged 50–69, not on HRT, 45 would normally be expected to develop breast cancer. The extra cases that would occur if they took HRT would be 2 per 1,000 after five years' use and 6 after ten years' use. Of those women aged 50–59 not taking HRT, 3 per 1000 would be expected to have a stroke over a five-year period. One extra case would occur in those taking HRT. Meanwhile, there was a reduction of four cases per 1,000 women aged 50–69 of colorectal cancer and a 9 cases per 1,000 reduction of hip fracture. So this black and white study was more of a muddy grey, with risks and benefits to be weighed. All the same, it firmly quashed the idea that HRT was cardio-protective.

The Committee on Safety of Medicines in Britain had taken a fairly sober view, albeit blown out of proportion by the media. This was not the case elsewhere in Europe. The head of the German Committee on Safety of Medicines likened HRT to thalidomide and raged about the way that a hormonal sickness had been created by the big pharmaceutical companies out of a natural phase of life. It wasn't a happy time for a woman on HRT.

The Million Women Study (MWS) began in 1996 and reported in *The Lancet* in August 2003. The MWS was an observational study which reviewed a wide range of different HRT regimens and administration routes (patches, gels, tablets and so on) among over a million women aged 50–64 who attended the NHS breast-screening programme and completed a questionnaire about HRT use. The analysis was based on 828,923 of them. The study was led by Professor Valerie Beral, one of Britain's most distinguished epidemiologists (scientists who study the distribution of disease determinants and risk amongst populations).

In sum, short-term use of HRT at the menopause results in very low additional risk of breast cancer. Longer use will give a higher risk, with the greatest risk being associated with implants and the least with patches. In real numbers, by the age of 65, one extra case of breast cancer per 1,000 women will have been caused by using oestrogen-only preparations for five years, or 5 extra cases if used for ten years. The comparable figures for combined preparations are 6 and 19. One curious finding was that an increased risk of breast cancer was seen after one year's use of combined HRT, but this was not seen in the WHI trial, where an increased risk was noted only after 3–4 years' use.

The MWS postulated (by extrapolating data) that HRT had been responsible for 20,000 additional cases of breast cancer over the past ten years in women aged 50–65. The reaction in the media was first, as you would expect, vilification of a profit-driven pharmaceutical industry, but there was also a significant under-current of this being women's own fault. If you try and hold back ageing, what do you expect? For comparison, using the same sort of extrapolation, amongst 50–65 year olds over the last ten years, 50,000 breast cancers have been caused by obesity and at least 16,000 breast cancers by alcohol intake, yet where is the censure from the media here?

The Committee on Safety of Medicines issued further advice on HRT in December 2003: it was to be used for relief of menopausal symptoms only. They also concluded that the risk/benefit ratio for osteoporosis was unfavourable and recommended other approaches. This recommendation flew directly in the face of information from the WHI study, which showed a considerable reduction in fracture rate, even among a group of women who were not at particular risk of osteoporosis.

What are ordinary women to make of all this information, some of which is contradictory and a lot of it alarming? The long and short of it is that some of the beneficial effects of HRT were exaggerated. HRT is absolutely not the heart-protecting medicine it was claimed to be and there is no justification for this use. Protection from Alzheimer's, once believed to be a benefit of HRT, is also unlikely. If you have miserable severe menopausal symptoms, HRT is an effective medicine to get you over the worst of them and there is no evidence that it causes harm with short-term use – benefits here outweigh risks. Thereafter, there is thinner ice and you have to let your own riskometer guide you, with what's important to you taking precedence. If you are at risk of osteoporosis, because of family or medical history, then you may feel comfortable trading knowledge of an increased risk of breast cancer for a reduction in something that you personally fear rather more. The evidence is that you should take it sooner rather than later, i.e. at the menopause, not years afterwards. HRT is emphatically not going to make you look or feel younger – that comes from inside and is as much about exercise, good food, not smoking and whose company you keep. My guess would be that a prescription for a toyboy who tells you how gorgeous you are before driving you wild with desire is probably more effective a rejuvenator than anything in pill form. When I mentioned this to a gynaecologist, he looked me up and down and said, 'We call that the noisy version of a testosterone patch.' Sign up for it now.

If you have local symptoms – dry vagina, urinary tract problems, a local agent would be first choice, rather than HRT pills. On the subject of pills, not all HRT preparations are the same. Lower doses of hormones can still be effective if given via patches or gels, whereas pills have to contain higher doses in order for sufficient active ingredient to survive breakdown by the liver. It is significant that these forms of HRT were those least associated with significant side effects in the Million Women Study.

Is HRT dead in the water? As a wonder protective drug – absolutely. It has taken fifty years for this hormone medication to come full circle and it is now back to exactly its first indications – symptomatic relief of severe menopausal symptoms. It is also effective for osteoporosis prevention if started early and maintained for a sufficient number of years, probably ten to fifteen, but may no longer be prescribed for this reason. The outrage from those who fear breast cancer has effectively ensured that the faint voices of the dispossessed crippled by osteoporosis have been drowned. Who cares about old ladies? Clearly not the CSM.

Don't misunderstand my message here. HRT was egregiously and sometimes wickedly over-promoted, partly by presenting menopause as a disease state. And medicalization of the menopausal state continues: a classic example is the way that Novo Nordisk promoted sales in Australia of their topical oestrogen, Vagifem, once HRT was under suspicion. In a textbook case of disease-mongering, they set up a website called www.whylovehurts to promote the more comfortable sex that women newly off HRT might have if they used the Vagifem product. They sent hairdressers scripted messages to use with clients, plus free capes for their salon, emblazoned with the web address.

To the disappointment of drug company shareholders, the market has returned to servicing a select few, not dosing the many. As a rule mass prescription does not suit the individual. The reverse is also true, that what is bad for the mass can still be right for certain individuals. This seems especially true of hormones, and it is easily forgotten that we are all individuals, with varying risk factors and highly varied hormone levels, and that each of us requires a personal hormone regime, not one designed for every-woman. For some women HRT is still the right choice.

My guess is that we will see increasing promotion of lower dose products and ones in which progesterone is substituted for proge-stogens (the natural rather than the synthetic), or of those that you dose level for yourself – in other words, adjusting the dose until you find the minimal level to relieve your symptoms.

Meanwhile, we may see increasing use of Selective Oestrogen Receptor Modulators (SERMS) which, as their name suggests, only act on oestrogen receptors in certain sites – for instance, not on womb-lining receptors (which you wouldn't want) but those like oestrogen receptors in bone. I suspect that there will be many more of these 'designer' types of HRT, which spare some tissues while targeting others.

Before leaving hormone replacement, let me issue a health warning. 'Natural' hormones are touted all over the internet as the answer to menopausal symptoms. Wild yam cream, for example, is promoted as containing natural hormones without the side effects: 'Stimulates the body's own production of hormones with natural progesterone.' 'Converts naturally to oestrogen and DHEA.' 'Prevents osteoporosis.' The only reason, these 'natural' hormone sites claim, that natural progesterone is not prescribed is because there's more money in patented synthetic sorts – progestins – even though they are dangerous. It's a seductive argument, but untrue.

For a start, the Mexican yam, *Dioscorea villosa*, is not actually a source of progesterone. The plant contains large amounts of something called diosgenin, which can be used to synthesize steroid hormones, including progesterone (a discovery which led to the first contraceptive pill). So if there is progesterone in wild yam cream (which is often doubtful), it's only there because it was synthesized in a lab first. Hardly the natural product you thought it was. Progesterone does indeed get converted in the body to other hormones (remember the description of steroid production as a conveyor belt, with progesterone being a steroid en route to oestrogen and testosterone) and that is why synthetic progestins are preferred to the natural variety, because they don't get instantly converted into other hormones. All hormones, synthetic or natural, have the ability to cause side effects.

Hormones are not available without prescription in Britain and quite rightly so. If there is enough hormone in a product for a company to make a medical claim, then it should be subject to all the stringent tests that are insisted on for medicines, including iteration of all possible side effects. The fact that these companies operate from offshore sites should tell you all you need to know. Will these people be around in twenty years' time when you discover that their product hasn't prevented osteoporosis? Quite. Don't go there.

There are some natural progesterone products available on prescription, including progesterone creams which do actually have enough progesterone in them to raise blood plasma levels of the hormone (unlike the products I have just mentioned). One is called Progest. It is said to be effective against osteoporosis, but there's no evidence whatsoever that these products have any effect in building bone. In fact, two separate trials, including one funded recently by the National Osteoporosis Society at the University of Southampton, have shown that they have no effect.

A vaginal progesterone gel (Crinone) is available to rub into the skin, rather than taking progestins with your oestrogen in tablet form. The gel can be used to protect the womb lining, though it has no licence for such use in the UK. It is also available as a pessary (Cyclogest). Both are reputable products only available on prescription but they do have the side effect of causing sleepiness. As you will remember from the chapter on pregnancy, progesterone in large doses can also be used as an anaesthetic. In the future, natural progesterone may be available as a nasal spray. Such developments mean that in future it may be possible to bring down the dose of hormones required for effect, thus minimizing side effects, and to tailor HRT to individual needs.

Eating for Your Hormones

Hormones are produced in response to change. The onset of winter or the appearance of a lover are two types of situation which get the brain sending out hormones – eating is another. There is a huge hormonal response *when* you eat: dozens of hormones are at work – insulin, glucagon, secretin – trying to bring you back to a state of equilibrium after you indulge. *What* you eat also influences hormone production and you can manipulate what you eat in order to manipulate your hormones. High-fat, low-fibre diets are associated with higher circulating levels of oestrogen – and we've already discovered that obesity is associated with later menopause. High fibre speeds up the clearance of oestrogen from the body. Severe constipation is associated with menstrual problems and with low circulating levels of oestrogen. There are also hormones in food, almost all derived from plants.

Plants have hormones just like humans. One plant hormone is the gas ethylene, which is involved in ripening. It's the invisible X-factor that infects green bananas with yellowness the instant a black banana is put next to them. Plants also contain substances which act like hormones when ingested by humans but which have no active hormone role in the plant. In the human gut they are transformed by intestinal bacteria to hormone-like compounds which produce an oestrogenic effect by binding to oestrogen receptors. Some may have an anti-oestrogenic effect, too, in that they compete with oestrogen for the receptor spaces. Collectively, they are called phytoestrogens and first came to attention some half a century ago when it was noticed that sheep grazing in clover pastures had oestrogen-related infertility. Their potential for preventing menopausal symptoms and also in mitigating breast cancer came to light when it was observed that in those countries, such as those in Asia, where large amounts of soy products (up to 100 mg per day) are consumed, the women had a lower rate of breast cancer than western women, who consume on average 5 mg per day.

There are three main groups of phytoestrogens: coumestans and isoflavonoids, which are very similar chemically, and lignans. Isoflavones are the largest group of natural isoflavonoids and are found in most plants of the pea family, including soy bean, clover, mung beans and alfalfa. The highest concentrations are found in a plant called kudzu root, followed by those in soy. There are several different forms of isoflavones in legumes: the most biologically active form is genistein. Coumestans are even more potent, and are found in bean shoots and sprouts, as well as in soy beans and spinach. Flaxseed (linseed) is the richest source of lignans followed closely by lingonberries, eaten by the Finns as part of a rye porridge meal, though lignans are also found in cereals.

Humans eat hundreds of milligrammes of phytoestrogens every day. To give you an idea of the scale of magnitude here, we eat 40 *million* times more natural oestrogen-mimicking products than we ingest synthetically produced ones. Phytoestrogens in food are a very common part of our diet.

Many women do not like taking hormones, or take them briefly and then find that they can't get on with them. If you do want to take HRT, accept that you may have to try several sorts before finding the one that's right for you. If you don't want to take hormones and have symptoms that are unpleasant, but not too serious, then you might want to consider upping your intake of phytoestrogens, or consider some of the herbal therapies. Black cohosh, a perennial plant of the buttercup family, is a native of North America and has the best evidence of oestrogenic activity. The dose is 8 mg of standardized extract per day in divided doses.

The effects of phytoestrogens are also subject to hype. If you have severe menopausal symptoms, you will not get the same level of relief from phytoestrogens as that given by HRT, although many women do say they work for milder problems. Even so, formal trials have been disappointing. Red clover proved no more effective than a placebo in preventing hot flushes, a multicentre trial reported in the *Journal of the American Medical Association* (*JAMA*) in July 2003. Nor is their overall activity proven. A recent study in 2004 (once again in *JAMA*, from the University of Utrecht) concluded that soya supplements did not protect bone mineral density or affect plasma lipids. Nevertheless, the flight into phytoestrogens continues apace, with two full bays of my local health-food store given over to 'phytoestrogens', with all sorts of claims made about their effects.

At this point, can I give you a further health (and wealth) warning? Just because something is natural, does not mean that those who manufacture it are automatically on the side of the angels. The big pharmaceutical companies are not the only ones making money out of hormones. HRT mayhem has created a gold rush for 'natural' products (most of which are processed chemically of course). There is almost no regulation in the supplement field and what enforcement there is, falls through a crack in the floor, somewhere between the Food Standards Authority and Trading Standards. There is acknowledged to be a particularly large placebo effect in relief of menopause symptoms, which means that it is easy for companies to make a killing at your expense. Moreover, where there is evidence of a dose-related response to a particular substance, many preparations fail to provide the appropriate dose, either because too little is put into a 'do-it-all' type of preparation or, and this is more common, simply because the product is not what it claims to be on the label. ConsumerLab (www.ConsumerLab.com) is a respected independent American organization which regularly tests supplements. It recently tested eighteen soy or red clover products and out of those five failed the test as they contained only between 50 and 80 per cent of the amount of active ingredient advertised on the label. I doubt the situation is any different in most of Europe.

If I were choosing a 'natural' product, I would avoid the combined sort (menopause formulas) and choose a single product from a reputable manufacturer. If it doesn't work for you, stop using it. I would also only consider using these products for relief of symptoms that you can monitor yourself – hot flushes, vaginal dryness etc. There are many claims that isoflavones will prevent bone loss but there are no long-term trials that support this assertion and the results of shorter trials are conflicting. One, from Denmark, noted bone *loss* when use of isoflavones was combined with a transdermal progesterone cream. A synthetic isoflavone, ipriflavone, has been under trial for some time and is available in some European countries and seems to preserve bone mass by increasing the effect of oestrogen.

If you are at risk of osteoporosis, stick to something proven – which means a prescription medicine. Osteoporosis isn't a hot flush, it's a condition which causes the death of tens of thousands of women each year and disables many more. If your life, not to mention quality of life, is potentially on the line, stick to something about which there is good evidence, not three twigs in a plastic bag costing an arm and a leg.

Is there harm associated with phytoestrogens? Soy milk, which enjoyed a brief surge of popularity as an alternative to infant formula, is currently not advised for babies as it has been found that the level of isoflavones known to cause menstrual disturbance in women is the same as that found in infant formula. The concern is particularly for baby boys, in whom disruption of normal hormonal-directed development may occur, resulting in an increased number of cases of testicular cancer, infertility or hypospadias. And yet there is no evidence of such problems in men in Japan or China; indeed, the high level of phytoestrogens consumed by men in Asia seems to protect them from cancers, in particular from prostate cancer. Phytoestrogens also have beneficial effects on heart health and it is worth making an effort to have more of them as you get older – but preferably from foods, not from supplements, as it is the combination of molecules in foods that appears to achieve some of the effects, rather than specific molecules alone.

Hormones and Cancer

BREAST CANCER AND OESTROGEN

So why does the risk of breast cancer rise so much after the menopause? Anything to do with hormones? Here is the truth about hormones and breast cancer – and it's not pretty. For the hormone women love for its softening, moistening and plumping effect is about to turn nasty.

Oestrogen is also the fuel for most breast cancers. About two thirds of all breast cancers are studded throughout with oestrogen receptors and are dependent on the hormone for growth.

Once upon a time, breast cancer was a relatively rare disease, except in nuns, and it was believed that it occurred if breasts were not used for their natural purpose. This has some truth in it. Oestrogen was first linked to breast cancer a century or so ago, when it was noted that removing the ovaries of women with breast cancer improved their chance of survival. Now it is known that naturally high levels of sex hormones, particularly oestrogens, double the risk of breast cancer for older women. Why should oestrogen have this effect?

We have seen how the menstrual cycle and the hormones that control it – oestrogen and progesterone – drive women's reproductive systems for the best part of four decades. You know yourself how your breasts alter in size with each cycle, going from perky insouciance just before a period to diving beneath your armpits when you lie down shortly after one. Breast tissue is one of the most active in the body, constantly being 'remodelled' each month in anticipation of a potential pregnancy. This activity is driven by both the reproductive hormones, but especially oestrogen.

Key 'target tissues' for oestrogen are the womb lining and breast, which are littered with receptors. As oestrogen docks with these receptors, it delivers its message loud and clear: divide. Oestrogen and the receptor travel together as a unit into the command centre of the cell, the nucleus. The unit instructs oestrogen-responsive genes to be switched on, and these then make the proteins that signal the cell to divide. A similar story applies to progesterone.

Every time your cells divide, your genetic material gets copied. The greater the number of cell divisions, the greater the chance of there being an error. It's a bit like photocopying a copy of a map – many, many copies later, a small detail may become too faint to read, sending you the wrong way. There is, however, a very efficient cellular housekeeping service, which ensures errors get corrected. This service becomes less efficient with age, meaning that some errors will get through. If the mistake affects one of the crucial genes that provide checks on cell growth, cells will suddenly proliferate uncontrollably, forming a cancer. So, that's why the greatest single risk factor for most cancers is age.

With breast cancer, it is not just chronological age that counts but, crucially, the length of time that your breast tissue has been exposed to both hormones, especially oestrogen, and all the cell division that this implies. That's why earlier age at first period or a late menopause are risk factors – more cycles means longer exposure to oestrogen than someone who started later. And having many children is also protective – every time you are pregnant, you stop ovulating for the best part of a year. The reverse of this is that, as with nuns, childless women are at greater risk because their breasts have not had a break from the relentless ebb and flow of hormones. All this is despite the fact that pregnancy subsumes women in a tidal wave of oestrogens, which might lead you to suppose that having many children would increase risk. But it doesn't and it seems that during pregnancy breast cells are protected in some way from damage and that, following birth, through irreversible changes which occur in the breast tissue, some degree of protection against breast cancer is conferred for life. This appears to be strengthened by breastfeeding. Much of the difference in breast cancer rates between developed and developing countries is related to breastfeeding and children, not just to diet as many people assume. It is estimated that if we had as many children as women in developing countries and breastfed for as long, our cumulative breast cancer incidence by the age of seventy would be halved to 2.7 per 100 women, an incidence not so dissimilar to that in developing countries of 2 per 100 by seventy.

Being obese after the menopause is a risk factor because the enzyme aromatase in fat cells can convert male hormones in the body to weak oestrogens, so that you continue your oestrogen exposure beyond the menopause. Remember that the breast is largely fat, so the breast also makes oestrogen post-menopausally, as well as being sensitive to it. Obesity has a double whammy effect for not only does it push up blood oestrogen levels, but also it reduces the amount of sex hormone binding globulins, the blood chaperones that keep steroid hormones in check. Work from the Endogenous Hormones and Breast Cancer Collaborative Group, led by the Cancer Research UK Epidemiology Unit in Oxford, established in 2002 that high circulating levels of oestrogens were associated with an increased risk of breast cancer in older women. High-fat, low-fibre western-style diets also increase risk because levels of circulating oestrogens are raised. This type of diet is the one most likely to make women obese.

Alcohol is a risk, again because it raises circulating levels of oestrogens, although the exact mechanism is unknown. Since heavy drinkers often have an unhealthy lifestyle generally (70 per cent of female heavy drinkers also smoke), it is not always easy to tease out the exact role of alcohol, although it seems that there is a dose response. The more you drink, the greater the risk.

The progression from a normal cell to one that is an out-of-control cancer cell consists of many steps. Some women are born with the first step already taken, in that they have a mutation in their genes – the best-known ones are BRCA1 and BRCA2 . Breast cancer genes are thought to cause about one in twenty breast cancers and typically can be seen at work in 'cancer families', where several relatives have had either breast or ovarian cancer, usually before the age of fifty.

Having told you about the risks, let's rank them to get an idea of how they compare. The way risk factors are compared is using relative risk (and this is often the figure you see quoted in the press) as you can see in the table below. A relative risk of 1 means no increase in risk. A risk of 1.5 increases risk by 50 per cent, a relative risk of 2 doubles it. This might sound a bit alarming but remember that relative risk means relative to people without the risk *of a similar age*.

RELATIVE RISK FACTORS FOR BREAST CANCER
(a relative risk of 1 is no risk)

Mother and sister affected	14
Age	8
Dense breasts	6
High plasma level oestrogens	5
Age at first birth over 35	1.9
More than 2 drinks a day	1.8
Never had children	1.6
Combined HRT	1.24

Let's say you are twenty-four and that eating zebras (to choose something totally false) has been discovered to have a relative risk of 2.0 with regard to breast cancer. The headlines for this might be 'Zebra meat doubles breast cancer risk', which is very alarming, particularly for you since you eat zebra daily. You might think, because you've heard that there is a 1 in 12 lifetime chance of breast cancer, that this means your risk is now 1 in 6, which would be very worrying indeed. It doesn't mean this.

To understand what a relative risk means for you, you have to know your risk of breast cancer right now, let's say you are twenty-four. Actually, before the age of twenty-five, risk of breast cancer is 1 in 200,000. A doubled relative risk *for you* means that instead of 1 per 200,000 women of your age being affected, in zebra eaters, it would be 2 per 200,000. Twice a small risk is still a small risk.

The woman most at risk from breast cancer is an old, fat, white nun, living in the West, who started her periods early, eats at McDonald's every day, and had a late menopause.

The biggest risk factor of all is being female, followed by age. There's not a lot you can do about either of those, nor about the genes you inherit. Apart from keeping yourself sober and trim there's not much on this table that is directly under your control, which is perhaps why something we *can* control (although right down at the bottom of the risk list) assumes such importance for us.

So oestrogen makes cells divide often and ups the chances of copying errors. Oestrogen can also tell breast cells how to respond to other hormones, such as progesterone, and growth factors. It has been discovered recently that breast tissue produces growth hormone and that cancerous cells make even more of it, transforming some breast cancers from relatively benign pussycats to ferocious tigers that break out and spread through the body (metastases). The mechanism is unknown as yet, but it wouldn't be a shock to discover that oestrogen had a hand in it.

Oestrogen is so far a proxy villain, engineering villainy rather than being caught red-handed, directly affecting cancer-causing processes in the cell. Current evidence suggests that sex hormones promote the growth of pre-existing cancers.

There are higher levels of oestrogens in breast tissue surrounding cancers than there are surrounding benign breast cysts. Something clearly is turning weak oestrogens into very potent ones. That enzyme, aromatase, is the culprit here, and aromatase inhibitors – things that prevent aromatase manufacturing oestrogen – are even more effective at preventing breast cancers than the oestrogen-blocking drugs, such as tamoxifen, which post-menopausal women are currently given. Because an aromatase inhibitor is more effective than an oestrogen-blocker, it suggests that aromatase activity is crucial in terms of increasing and enhancing the effects of oestrogen. This all sounds gloomy. Your own hormones turning on you – hormones with such widespread and powerful effects too. The good news about this is that hormonal therapies – or should I say, anti-hormonal therapies – are the great success story of breast cancer.

The drugs that block oestrogen receptors stop oestrogen latching on to breast cancer cells and making them grow. Tamoxifen is the best known and is used after surgery (adjustment therapy) in those women that have oestrogen receptor-positive cancers: one tablet is taken a day for five years. It is thought to be responsible for a good half of the drop in deaths from breast cancer in post-menopausal women. For such women, aromatase inhibitors like letrozole and exemestane are now being evaluated in large clinical trials. These drugs probably confer a small but absolute increase in survival compared with tamoxifen but data about their side effect profile (for instance, their effect on bones) is still incomplete and they are not yet currently licensed for adjuvant treatment in the UK.

Another way of stopping oestrogen is to remove the ovaries or stop them working with radiotherapy (ablation). This is clearly an irreversible strategy and is only suitable for women past the menopause. A potentially reversible way of achieving the same effect is to use something called a pituitary down regulator. The best known of these drugs is goserelin (Zoladex). It stops production of luteinising hormone and follicle stimulating hormone (which, as you will recall is what tells the ovary to produce oestrogen). In effect it brings on a premature menopause.

A final word on breast cancer. No doubt you have heard some very alarming figures about the increase in breast cancer. Breast cancer incidence (which reflects the numbers of women diagnosed with breast cancer, not those who die from it) increased in the UK all through the 1980s, from 79 per 100,000 in 1980 to 114 per 100,000 just twenty years later. It reached a peak in 1992. Our genes don't change in such a short space of time, so the logical conclusion is that there is something about our modern lifestyle which is causing this huge increase in numbers of women with breast cancer.

Much of the increase since 1988 has occurred in women aged 50–64, who had been invited to attend the national screening programme started at this time. In other words, women who previously had died of something else, or who had tumours that never became invasive, were now being spotted and were being added to the breast cancer statistics, pushing up the incidence rate dramatically.

Another reason for the increased numbers is that we are an ageing population: more older women, more breast cancer. But the figures have age ironed out of them using a system called age weighting. In Britain, for example, comparing breast cancer incidence in Eastbourne, which has a high number of retired people, with an area which has a lot of young families would be an unfair comparison, so the figures are adjusted using mathematical formulas in order to compare areas on the same basis. Recently the age weightings in the US have been revised – they had not been changed since 1970. Nassau County, for instance, had an incidence of 112.8 per 100,000. New age weighting meant an incidence rate of 136 per 100,000. There were exactly the same number of breast cancer cases, just a different age weighting formula. In other words, figures aren't always what they seem and you always need to be sure that you are comparing like with like before jumping too quickly to a conclusion.

Age apart, there is still an increase and some of it is readily explainable by what we already know about breast cancer risk factors. For instance, earlier puberty, obesity, greater alcohol intake amongst women, the marked trend for later pregnancy and fewer children, have all increased incidence rates. That leaves about 5 per cent of the recent rise unexplained, which is a cause for concern, but not for panic and self-flagellation.

PROSTATE CANCER AND TESTOSTERONE

Men have the same problems with testosterone as women do with oestrogen – friend becomes foe over time. The prostate is a troublesome muscular gland that sits below the bladder, surrounding the tube leading from the bladder to the outside (urethra). It makes prostatic fluid, an important component of semen, and then squeezes it out at ejaculation (something which incidentally stops men peeing at orgasm). The gland is troublesome because it increases in size with age, the growth being testosterone-dependent. The body is normally good at controlling testosterone so that the gland doesn't get too big even during the testosteronefest that is adolescence. The control system appears to be less effective with age, because, even with less testosterone in the system, the prostate gets bigger than it should. This condition – benign prostatic hyperplasia or BPH – is usually seen from middle age onwards. Because the urethra effectively goes right through the middle of the prostate gland, it can get squashed when the gland becomes enlarged, causing poor urine flow, and many urinary problems for older men. The prostate gland, for reasons that are unknown, also seems prone to becoming cancerous and almost all men reaching extreme old age will die with prostate cancer, though not of it.

Prostate cancer *can* become aggressive, however, and is the cause of death in 10,000 men each year in Britain. Just as in breast cancer, one of the ways to choke its growth is to starve it of the hormone it needs. Just like breast cancer, pituitary down regulators like goserelin can be used to shut down luteinising hormone, which is telling the testicles to produce testosterone. There are also anti-androgens, which perform the same sort of job as tamoxifen. And there are oestrogens. Stilboestrol is a synthetic oestrogen which fools the body into thinking that it must switch off testosterone production. The side effects for men undergoing hormonal therapy can be substantial, and include loss of libido, impotence and hot flushes. This is why hormonal therapy is usually only offered when the cancer has spread. Even when the cancer is no longer in the prostate, it is still driven by testosterone, with many receptors for it, wherever it has lodged. You might be thinking at this point that we'd be better off without our reproductive hormones. Yet the benefits still outweigh the risks that they inflict on us in later years.

We have talked about the crash of hormones in women, but not yet discussed the male equivalent. Is there a male andropause? The question of whether men experience a 'change of life' because of falling hormone levels as they age is controversial. We are certainly all familiar with male mid-life crisis. The sudden conversion to black T-shirts, rather than shirt and tie, the soft top car that appears in the driveway, air guitar to Led Zeppelin and the pursuit of women young enough to be their daughters. Is it a hormone crash or just a sudden realization that there are not enough years left to do everything they ought to have done in their youth? A medical crisis requiring treatment – or part of life's rich tapestry?

That it might be a medical matter is not a new concept. In 1813, a paper by Sir Henry Halford was read at the Royal College of Physicians. In it he talked of a disease affecting men aged between fifty and seventy-five: 'Sometimes the disorder comes on so gradually and insensibly that the patient is hardly aware of its commencement … in process of time his appetite become seriously impaired, his nights are sleepless … his face becomes visibly extenuated or perhaps acquires a bloated look. He suspects he has a fever.' Sir Henry had no suggestions as to treatment other than warm purgatives and local evacuations. (No, I don't know what they involved either, but fear the worst.)

A hundred years later, the word 'climacteric', previously applied only to women and the menopause, was being used for the first time of men. In 1909 Archibald Church, a famous neurologist of his day, published an article on 'Nervous and mental disturbances of the male climacteric', dealing with symptoms that he claimed had a monthly rhythm in men and of the 'minor psychoses and neurotic disturbances of men aged between fifty and sixty-five'. He claimed that criminal behaviour in men peaked in the sixth decade. Certainly it's the age at which men start to dress criminally.

Organotherapy was of course the solution. In 1916, the sexologist Max Marcuse from Berlin was treating male climacteric patients with his own preparations – Testikulin, Testogan or Hormin – prepared no doubt from testicles, although their exact contents were like the Coca-Cola formula, a secret that Mr Marcuse guarded closely. It's unlikely that they had any effect. The unlucky ones were subjected to faradization – given a bolt of electricity to the prostate gland – which sounds eye-wateringly awful.

The first standardized preparations of male hormones appeared in the early 1930s. This was relatively late, a reflection of the technical difficulties, but also of the beliefs spawned by the gland-grafters that male ageing could be restored only by implanting donor testicular tissue (rather than an extract) into the host. The gland-grafters (not to mention the organotherapists before them) had created an atmosphere in which all hormones, and particularly testosterone, were associated with quackery, and those companies that had testosterone products were unwilling to market them aggressively, fearing that if they did, they would be damned by association. When testosterone was first brought to market, by the Dutch company Organon, it was prescribed for male urinary complaints, and marketed through urologists in a deliberate attempt to distance the product from the dubious activities of the rejuvenators.

The hormone preparations of this time were, as noted previously, drugs looking for medical diseases to treat. Sexual problems were not considered a medical problem at the time, with very few men even admitting that they had them. Although there was an interest in the male climacteric, the pharmaceutical companies of the time wanted to project themselves as being science-based, and were wary of doing anything that might possibly tar them with some of the wilder claims of the organotherapists.

Organon produced the first standardized testicular extract, Hombreol, obtained from bulls' testicles, in 1931, later switching to urine as a source, obtained from thousands of Dutch soldiers at a nearby barracks. It was at this time that so-called paradoxical hormone treatment began, in which male hormones were given to women and, rather less frequently, female hormones given to men. Prior to this time, the sexes and their hormones were strictly delineated. Then it was discovered that, counter-intuitively, the testicles of stallions, rather than ovaries of mares, were the richest source of the oestrogen, oestrone, while androgens were found in quantity in female as well as male urine. Later it was realized that sex steroids come not just from the ovaries or testes but from the adrenal gland too. Nowadays testosterone is advocated for loss of libido in older women. It was synthetic testosterone's availability that prompted its wider application – especially for age-related sexual problems – when it first appeared in 1935. This time, the hormone 'drug' appeared to have found its 'disease' – sexual difficulties.

By 1939, there was alarm from the Council on Pharmacy and Chemistry, who thundered in the *Journal of the American Medical Association*: 'Within the past few months extravagant claims for the action of the male sex hormone testosterone have appeared in professional and lay publications ... it is the Council's belief that many claims for it have been grossly exaggerated.' War intervened, but still the testosterone fires were raging. The *Journal of the American Medical Association* felt it necessary to write a dampening editorial in 1942: 'Brochures circulated by pharmaceutical manufacturers depict the woeful course of aging man. None too subtly, these brochures recommend that male hormonal substance, like a veritable elixir of youth, may prevent or compensate for the otherwise inevitable decline. What of the postulated occurrence of a climacteric in men?' What indeed?

The 'male climacteric' is not a phrase that finds much favour amongst the public – how do you pronounce it for a start? The word 'andropause' finds equal disfavour among doctors because it implies a biology in men that is comparable to that in women, in whom there is a precipitous fall in hormones, a 90 per cent drop from oestrogen pre- to post-menopause, for instance which is certainly not the case in men. Perhaps a new phrase is needed: the current favourite seems to be androgen deficiency in ageing males or ADAM.

It is clear that testosterone falls with age, but nowhere near as dramatically as oestrogen does in women. By the age of eighty, the blood free testosterone of a man is about half what it was at twenty. This is not simply caused by a decrease in production of testosterone but by a well-documented increase in the steroid 'chaperones' in the blood, the sex hormone binding globulins. Free testosterone begins to decline about the age of thirty with a consistent decrease of about 2 per cent a year thereafter. This decline is hastened in particular by obesity but also by diseases such as heart failure and lung cancer, inflammatory disease, and by heavy drinking. There seems to be an alteration in the rhythms of testosterone production, with the usual night-time elevations reduced. If blood levels of testosterone fall, the body would normally ramp up its gonadotrophin releasing hormone, so generating more luteinising hormone, which in turn stimulates the testicles to produce more testosterone. As men age, the hypothalamus seems to become selectively deaf as far as low testosterone levels are concerned, with all parts of the system less efficient than they were. The siren call of gonadotrophin releasing hormone (which controls testosterone production) is somehow less compelling than it was. It appears that the testes, too, have become deaf to the calls for action arriving on their doorstep.

There is a lot of debate about the prevalence of low testosterone in older men and what is a 'significant' decrease. The situation is bedevilled by arguments about exactly how you measure testosterone and also by the fact that there is no consistency about levels at which symptoms appear – what's low for one man is perfectly fine for another. The defining level for diagnosis of hypogonadism (a medical condition in which testosterone production is regarded as deficient) is a total testosterone of less than 8.7 nanomoles per litre

– by this measure, less than 10 per cent of older men are testosterone deficient. Other studies use reference levels of 10.4 or even 11 and find by that measure, 20 or even 30 per cent are deficient. The long and short of it is that you can create as big a population as you like of 'deficient' men by playing about with the definition of 'low'. When we talk about 'low', are we talking low as in low for sixty, or low compared to a twenty year old, which would include three quarters of older men?

You might ask whether testosterone decreases because it is no longer required for the fathering of babies. In fact, although fertility declines in men with age, they can, and do still father babies when in their eighties and nineties. So, the fall in testosterone seems to be a consequence of ageing, not a cause of it. Thus technically speaking, male fertility ends with death, and in that sense there is no comparison between andropause and menopause because women continue to live beyond their fertility, while for men, the ending of fertility is likely to be a lethal condition.

The gradual decline in testosterone does affect fantasies and sexual thoughts, which become much less common as men age. Thinking of sex every six seconds is definitely a pursuit of the young. However, it should be said, such is the variation between men that some men will be enjoying sexual thoughts even as they knock on the pearly gates. By the way, it is a myth that many older men die *in flagrante*. Statistically, golf is much more dangerous.

Perhaps the decline in libido is for the best, because impotence is a major and deeply frustrating problem of ageing, affecting about half of all men over forty. It is tempting to attribute the declining frequency of sex with age to decreasing levels of testosterone, but although impotence can be caused by low testosterone (hypogonadism), it is an uncommon cause (less than one in twenty). A much more usual reason for erectile dysfunction is anything that affects blood flow to the penis, thus disturbing the elegant hydraulic system which powers its tumescent activity, such as smoking, atherosclerosis or diabetes. Circulating levels of testosterone in older men experiencing erection problems are normally well above those required for a normal sexual response and, sadly, restoring testosterone levels will not rejuvenate a penis flagging because its blood supply is weak compared to that of its glory days.

To my mind, age is never an acceptable excuse for tackle that doesn't do what it should, and men should no more accept it than women should. Women need to be close to have sex, but for men sex is the route to closeness. If sex is taken away, a hugely important reservoir of comfort and self-esteem is removed. It is not surprising that men, believing that testosterone is the route back to the comforts as well as the thrill of sex, hanker after it so much.

What is certain is that decreasing levels of testosterone are associated with decreased muscle, thinner bones, reduced body hair, skin thickness, cognition, endurance, mood and well-being. Who wouldn't hanker when told that testosterone can improve sexual interest, erectile function, muscle mass, mood and body hair – which is what is promised in a leaflet from the US-based Hormone Foundation, supported by an unrestricted grant from Solvay Pharmaceuticals US, makers of Androgel, a testosterone preparation.

So should replacement testosterone be offered to men? Is there any point in pouring androgens into a system which has become less responsive to them, perhaps even to the point of no response at all? There have been many poor pieces of research in this field, but a careful and important study by Peter Snyder and his team from the University of Pennsylvania in 1999 showed clear, although modest benefits over a three-year period for older men given 6 mg per day via a patch, with striking dose-dependent testosterone effects which were inversely proportional to plasma testosterone at the start of the study. In other words, those that had the lowest levels to start off with, benefited the most. This was a short-term study, however. There are major concerns with longer term safety, principally that increasing testosterone will result in prostate enlargement (leading to urinary problems) and accelerate prostate cancer. The data on increased heart disease is equivocal. High red-blood cell counts and behavioural problems are also a risk. The studies are rather opaque on what these behavioural difficulties might be – I've always imagined that it is sixty-five year olds having teenage temper tantrums rather than sixty-five year olds going out to buy a Harley Davidson. What's more, it is a sad irony that one of the symptoms of prostate cancer and of coronary heart disease is erectile dysfunction – thus the very elixir taken to spur a flagging member on has the potential to cause precisely that same problem.

Another concern is that the focus on testosterone may distract from proper assessment and treatment of the underlying health problems that have prompted men to seek help. For those men that are genuinely hypogonadal, constantly fatigued, with testicular atrophy, fading bones and a low libido, there is surely a place for testosterone. What is truly concerning is how ADAM has suddenly become a medical disease, requiring aggressive treatment. It is noticeable, too, that the 'low' number is inching its way upwards. At the time of writing this book, yet another company announced that it would be entering the androgen market. Meanwhile, other pharma companies (and not just those that don't list androgens among their products) are becoming alarmed by the way in which testosterone is being marketed. They fear a disaster ahead, and they are right in that apprehension.

While women are concerned about risk – the flight from HRT after the Million Women Study was published is but one illustration – men are much less risk averse. Three years of hot sex and then you die? Fine, lead me to it, seems to be the attitude of some older men. They seem to think, in this testosterone-induced nirvana, that one day they will be felled by a massive heart attack while pleasuring some nubile woman, and out they'll go, the envy of their mates. Life isn't like that. A long miserable decline into chronic ill-health is more likely and it is at this point that men will finally wake up and realize that they were misled. Yes, it was their hormones (or the remants of them) that led them by the nose, but they were actively seduced too. This is also the point – when the miseries of prostate cancer or chronic heart disease become intrusive and all pervading, men will turn around and sue the drug companies. If this were a no-risk exercise, then I'd be manning the barricades on behalf of men, but testosterone, as we've seen time and time again, is a very powerful hormone and the risks of taking it are considerable. Men need to be protected from themselves. Fat chance.

My prediction is this: I think that we will see the pattern of HRT repeated with testosterone-replacement therapy. Early enthusiasm, tempered by the exposure of dangers, followed by the development of designer testosterones (in the way that we have had selective oestrogen receptor modulators (SERMS) like raloxifene for osteoporosis), which can deliver the good things, but not the bad. Unlike HRT, expect to see these products as street drugs, peddled as Viagra is today, to young men on street corners, not just prescribed to older men in doctors' waiting rooms. For surely, you can never have too much of a good thing?

So here ends the story of how our hormones turn on us. We are still better off with them than without them and perhaps, having read this chapter, you have a better understanding of their malignant power, as well as their benefits. One final observation: Brown-Séquard, the pioneer of hormones, brilliantly brought us the concept of internal secretion, and then with his youth elixirs brought testosterone into disrepute, making it a no go hormone thereafter for science-based business. But for this, the pharmaceutical giants might not have concentrated on hormonal products for women but started with those for men. This could have changed the course of medical history.

CHAPTER SEVEN

DO HORMONES MAKE YOU FAT?

When I was a child growing up in Portsmouth, the naval town on the south coast, and we saw someone who was grossly obese, my mother would say pityingly, in a knowing stage whisper, 'Trouble with their glands, dear.' In those days Portsmouth was full of sailors of all nationalities and anyone who was very fat was unusual. Now, when I go back to my home town forty years later, the sailors have all gone and people who are very overweight are so common as to be unremarkable. The attitude to these heavyweights has also changed. They are no longer the subject of pity, but of a kind of loathing. Fat today says greedy, slothful and self-indulgent. As I will show you, hormones and obesity and intimately bound together. Trouble with your glands is indeed part of the obesity equation, including a gland that has only in the last decade been discovered to be secreting hormones – fat itself.

The world is facing an epidemic of obesity. In the UK alone, over a thousand people a week die prematurely from the complications of obesity. Being obese doubles your chances of getting bowel and breast cancer, ups the likelihood of osteoarthritis, especially of knees and hips, and causes Type 2 diabetes, hypertension, strokes and heart attacks. We are big, and getting bigger. In fact, according to the 2004 House of Commons Health Select Committee Report on Obesity, the proportion of the UK population that is obese has grown fourfold in the last twenty-five years, the fastest rate of increase in Europe. In Nordic countries there has been no such change, although it may be beginning.

Contrary to belief, we don't actually eat that much more than people did fifty years ago in energy terms, although the proportion of our fuel that we obtain from fats and sugars has increased. Actually, according to latest data, we eat less. The main difference is that we exercise much less. There are far fewer manual jobs. We now go to work to sit down, and go home to be active. We work further away from home, which means that we don't walk or cycle to get to work any longer. If you live in the US, cities are ribbons along highways with seemingly no means of walking anywhere. In Britain, children are no longer expelled on to freezing games pitches five times a week. They may do as little as forty minutes of compulsory games a week – instead of five hours a week, with a few more at the weekend, as their parents did.

In the past, and in some societies still, being fat was associated with wealth and was an aspiration. Today, being fat is linked with lower incomes, a higher divorce rate and with increased rates of depression and suicide. Patients being treated for obesity report that they would prefer to be blind or deaf than to be obese again. In 1997, a widely reported study by psychologists revealed that 15 per cent of women and 11 per cent of men would be prepared to sacrifice five years of life if only they could die slim. Discrimination against the obese is pervasive. The psychologist J. R. Staffieri, in what has become a classic study of childhood stereotypes, reported young children describing silhouettes of an overweight child with words like lazy, dirty, stupid, cheat and liar. The view of the obese by the lean is that they have done it to themselves and there is little or no sympathy for them.

Being obese would have been bad news for the evolving human. It would have meant not being agile enough to run away from danger and being too fat would also have brought additional dangers from disease like heart attack or stroke. On the other hand, being too thin was equally bad news. For women, it would have meant no pregnancies, since this depends on having at least 18–22 per cent of body fat, and for both sexes insufficient fat reserves to cope with periods of hardship would have meant a high likelihood of death by starvation. Thus having just the right amount of fat – neither too much, nor too little – is crucial to our survival and the body has an extraordinarily complex system devoted to keeping weight (and thus body fat) stable, no matter what.

Despite the variations in our day to day food intake and rate of exercise, most of us do remain pretty much the same size. Even if we diet, we find ourselves inexorably putting weight back on until we are once again the 'right' weight. It's a shame our bodies and our mirrors disagree on what 'right' is. By the time we reach old age, we are all heavier than we were in youth, but only by a stone or so, which creeps on insidiously as we age, although this isn't the case in more primitive societies. To see true weight stability in action, you only have to see teenage boys troughing. Their food intake would shame a lumberjack, but despite them lazing about like beached seals in their bedrooms, most (but not all) of them appear to stay the same size. This all points to there being some central weight thermostat, an idea that we will explore in this chapter. By now, you will not be surprised to hear that it's a system driven by hormones – although they, of course, are only responding to our lifestyle.

The body is not much concerned by whether we can fit in size 12 or size 10 jeans. Its overriding need is to maintain a state of internal constancy, no matter what is thrown at it. Food intake, running a marathon, stress, cold, heat, thirst – whatever the challenge from the outside, on the inside the body's challenge is to respond while keeping things exactly the same – or within a very narrow new range set by our activity. This internal constancy is essential in order to run body functions at maximal efficiency. Hormones are vital to this process, for they are constantly shuttling back and forth, carrying vital bits of information about internal change or, indeed, external changes, and being sent out with instructions to get things back on track. The relationships between the many hormones involved in this system are fantastically complex. We'll concentrate here on those involved in the regulation of energy balance and of appetite. Energy that is excess to requirements is stored as fat.

Thyroid

Because people understand that those with underactive thyroids become fat and those with overactive thyroid glands thin, they think that the thyroid is in charge of fat control and it must be a major part of the obesity story. This is not the case.

The thyroid is in charge of temperature control and has a major influence on energy metabolism. Its hormones can speed up the pace of metabolism, making more chemical reactions take place in the body. A faster speed creates more heat and a higher body temperature. Slow it all down and the body temperature drops. Extra metabolic speed means that more food is burned for heat energy and there is less to be stored. As a consequence fat stores may decrease, and your body interprets this, as we shall see later, as starvation, prompting hormones to be dispatched to sharpen appetite.

The deficiency and excess states of thyroid hormone are well known. Too little and people (particularly older women) become slow and lethargic, they put on lots of weight, frequently becoming obese, they feel the cold and have dry skin. Too much and people become mile-a-minute twitchy bags of nerves. Often these people have thyroid eye disease, in which typically the eyes bulge. Thyroid hormone has effects throughout the body, particularly on the muscles needed for heart and lung function.

When this was discovered, there was a vogue, particularly in the 1920s and 1930s, for advertising thyroid extract pills as the anti-fat solution. Those taking them had a nasty habit of dying. With too much thyroid, muscle tissue gets consumed for energy, leaving people feeble and gaunt, and tremor sets in as nerves become more and more excitable. Heart failure was common.

Insulin and Diabetes

So if thyroid isn't the hormone of fat, how about insulin, the hormone of plenty?

Over the last fifty years, the incidence of Type 2 diabetes (in which too much insulin is produced) has rocketed, in parallel with the incidence of obesity. This is despite us eating less – often a lot less – than our parents and grandparents. Some scientists believe that the availability of refined foods, particularly the increase in the amount of fat from diet from about 25 per cent to the present 35 per cent, plus the lack of physical activity, causes changes in muscle which are responsible for the development of Type 2 diabetes and obesity.

In diabetics, levels of glucose are higher than they should be in the blood, either because it is not taken up rapidly enough into tissues such as muscle, heart and fat, or because too much glucose is produced by the liver.

Glucose is a primary fuel for many tissues, and for the brain and nervous system, which powers through about 120 grams of glucose a day, it is almost essential. In extremis, it will make do with a substitute derived from fat, known as ketone bodies, but if it is doing this, then you are likely to be pretty much in extremis yourself – either starving, or dying from insulin-dependent diabetes.

The proper name for diabetes is *diabetes mellitus*, which means literally 'sweet fountain', referring to the fact that a high concentration of glucose in the blood spills over into the urine and gives it a characteristic malty smell. It is said that doctors from ancient times detected diabetes by a taste test – whether this is apocryphal or not is unknown.

Diabetes is in fact two separate diseases with the same end result: raised blood glucose (hyperglycaemia). The first, insulin-dependent diabetes, is an autoimmune disease, which starts early in life, often in childhood, in which the patches of tissue in the pancreas that produce insulin are destroyed. Normally insulin is made in response to the appearance in blood of glucose, which has been absorbed from the gut following a meal. Carbohydrates like potatoes and bread release most glucose when digested.

By far the greater number of people suffering from diabetes have the sort known as Type 2 or late-onset diabetes. This, as its name suggests, appears in later life, after forty usually, although it can occur at a younger age than this in some communities, for example in Indians living in Britain. Here there is not a lack of insulin – far from it, for insulin levels are higher than normal – but rather an inability of the normally insulin-sensitive tissues like muscle and the liver to respond to it.

So how does insulin work, in a normal, healthy person? After a meal, rising levels of glucose cause insulin to be secreted. Insulin drives glucose into muscle tissue (which makes up about a third of the total body weight in a lean person), including that of the heart (which is a big lump of muscle) where it will be stored as glycogen, the precursor fuel needed to power muscle exertion. Insulin also prompts a switch from the liver generating glucose – a process which ensures that between meals the blood concentrations of glucose can be kept more or less constant – to packing glucose away into storage depots. Glucose is stored either as glycogen, a carbohydrate fuel, or as triglycerides, fats similar to those found in olive oil, corn oil or lard. Significantly, for our obesity tale, insulin also drives glucose into body fat, where it is stored as triglycerides.

If insulin is not present at all – as in insulin-dependent diabetes, then muscle tissue cannot build up the reserves of glycogen fuel that it needs during exertion. The effect of no insulin is to put the body in a state which is very similar to starvation. In desperation, it responds by breaking down the triglycerides stored in fat which then, as fatty acids, can be used as an alternative fuel by muscle and heart – but not by the brain which, as we have seen, needs glucose.

In Type 2 diabetes, there is at first no shortage of insulin. In fact, early in the disease, there is more than usual. Yet, despite the insulin making its presence known in the muscle tissue, the muscle remains deaf to insulin's messages, no matter how many are sent, and does nothing to stimulate the uptake of glucose or the storage of glycogen.

Another hormone which comes from the pancreas, in cells which live very near to those which make insulin, is glucagon. Whereas insulin is the hormone of plenty, glucagon is the hormone of scarcity: so when glucose is taken into the blood from the intestine during digestion of starchy foods, insulin is secreted and glucagon secretion is inhibited. During the night, when there is nothing left in your gut to absorb, glucagon secretion increases and insulin secretion is inhibited. As we've just seen, if insulin levels are low, the liver switches into generating glucose mode once more, a process called gluconeogenesis. In healthy people, insulin and glucagon have a reciprocal relationship with one another, a bit like those wonderful Swiss weather houses, where as Mrs Sun comes out, Mr Rain disappears – and vice versa. In Type 2 diabetes, however, this relationship becomes altered so that glucagon levels are often high despite insulin secretion being high too.

So what's the relationship between being fat and sedentary and Type 2 diabetes? The argument goes something like this: normally muscle uses a large amount of fat to sustain low-level activities. For instance, when we get up in the morning and have a shower and make breakfast, we are almost entirely fuelled by fat. That's the reason why early-morning exercise, before breakfast, is best for fat burning.

In physically active people this fat mostly comes from stores within the muscle itself. However, in unfit people, fat gets stored in the wrong place in the muscle, so during early-morning exercise most of the fat has to be taken from the bloodstream instead, which although it sounds like it might be a good thing, isn't. This wrongly stored fat is already a cause of problems, because in order to store it, glucose has had to be pushed out – a bit as if you'd flung out everything in a cupboard to make room for something new. If glucose isn't being used in the muscle it accumulates in the blood, raising blood sugars and prompting the release of insulin. We've seen that if you have Type 2 diabetes your muscles are no longer listening to the messages being sent by insulin. So when you have breakfast in the morning, the glucose released as your cornflakes are being digested causes a higher rise in blood glucose than in a normal person, because it is not being taken up into muscle.

So here you are: you're unfit, so your muscles aren't storing glucose properly; you have high blood levels of glucose; insulin is produced in greater and great quantity in order to get shot of that glucose, but your muscles are now deaf to insulin's exhortations to take in glucose. Meanwhile, although your muscle has become insulin-resistant, for a while fat has no such problem – it retains its insulin sensitivity for some time and therefore helpfully takes up glucose at insulin's insistence, maintaining glucose stores in fat. Meanwhile, the liver also succumbs to insulin resistance, just like the muscles and, when soon after a meal insulin would normally shut down its glucose-generating operation and go into glucose-storing mode, it continues to produce glucose at a supernormal level in those with Type 2 diabetes throughout the day. So it's a vicious escalator in which being unfit and sedentary sends glucose levels up, tissues become insulin-resistant, and your body helpfully stuffs all that extra glucose away as fat.

It's not all the fault of hormones, however. For Type 2 diabetes it seems that there is a strong genetic predisposition to the development of high insulin levels, insulin-resistance and other features of the so-called 'metabolic syndrome' such as the tendency to store excess fuel as fat, the development of osteoarthritis and high blood pressure. Some suggest that those who possessed such a gene in the past were at an advantage in times of food scarcity, for they put on weight quickly. Today they are at a disadvantage. The underlying message is clear, however: lack of exercise plus genetic predisposition plus too much food equals Type 2 diabetes.

We've looked at thyroid hormones, we've looked at insulin, but still haven't got to the core of why some people eat a lot and others don't. Let me now introduce you to the Fat Controller.

The Fat Controller and the Hormone of Starvation?

There are many hormones which are involved in the control of appetite and satiety. Satiety is the feeling of being full up. These hormones are all part of that weight thermostat, which has three components: incoming signals that tell the brain about the body's nutritional state – too fat, too thin, hungry, full up; a controller (the hypothalamus in the brain); and outgoing signals that control metabolism and coordinate food intake such as a sharpening or dulling of appetite.

For many years, although it seemed obvious that there must be blood-borne messengers reporting nutritional state to the brain, no one could find them. It was assumed that it must be insulin. Indeed, if insulin is injected directly into the hypothalamus of rats, they eat less food. The evidence that this was a factor in humans was less than compelling, for people with Type 2 diabetes gain rather than lose weight when they first start to use insulin.

The breakthrough came just a decade ago. In December 1994, the front cover of *Nature* showed two sleek, lean mice on one side of a balance, failing to shift just one fat mouse on the other side. It sat there, a gargantuan fur ball, looking more like a wind-up toy than a real animal. Soon the fat mouse was a magazine cover story right across the world.

These roly-poly creatures were three times heavier than normal mice, and also had five times the body fat content of their leaner companions. They had a double defect in a gene called ob (as in *ob*ese) and were called *ob/ob* mice. Within a year it had been discovered that the protein product of this gene was a hormone called leptin, from the Greek *leptos*, meaning thin, and that it was predominantly manufactured in adipose tissue – fat. These mice, with their double mutation, produced no leptin at all. When in 1995 Jeffrey Friedman and Stephen Burley of Rockefeller University, New York, announced in *Science* magazine that injections of leptin had reduced body weight in these ob mice by 30 per cent after just two weeks' treatment, there was uproar. Could it really be so simple? Could this newly discovered hormone be *the* anti-obesity drug?

But it wasn't that simple. If fat cells produce leptin, surely people who have lots of fat must have lots of leptin – and tests showed that, pretty much, they did. So it was no good giving them more. One drug company, Amgen, did run a clinical trial just in case, to double-check. As it happens, there were a few people who lost weight – but there was no effect at all on the vast majority.

Meanwhile, scientists searched in vain for a similar gene in humans but without success. Then a team from the MRC Metabolic Disorders Unit in Cambridge, led by Professor Stephen O'Rahilly and Dr Sadaf Farooqi, reported the remarkable case of two cousins. O'Rahilly has a reputation for being a master mystery solver, the man to whom perplexed physicians send all their most difficult cases – and these two children were certainly that. They were both of normal weight at birth, but from the age of about four months developed an insatiable hunger. They ate far more than their siblings and a great deal more than their parents. In a test breakfast, the two year old consumed an adult's entire day's calories in one sitting and would still have eaten more. The pair scavenged for food in rubbish bins, ate fish fingers, still frozen, direct from the freezer, broke open padlocked cupboards to get at flour. Their hunger was all-consuming. It was, as Farooqi says, 'way beyond gluttony'. They behaved as if they were starving, yet both were grossly obese. The elder child, a girl, then aged ten, weighed 13½ stone. Despite having liposuction and surgery she was no longer able to walk. Her cousin, a boy of two, already weighed nearly 5 stone and seemed destined to follow his cousin. All other members of the immediate family were of normal weight.

The children came from a Bengali family and the father and

mother of each child were first cousins. Marriage between cousins, so called consanguineous marriage, is not culturally acceptable, and sometimes actually illegal in the West, but is extremely common in many parts of the world, where marrying 'in' is regarded as both normal and an important way of consolidating family wealth and influence. We all carry abnormal genes, but luckily, because we carry our genes in pairs and the normal one's instructions normally trump those of the abnormal one, their effects are not revealed. A close genetic relationship between parents, as with a marriage between first cousins, means a greater likelihood of their children inheriting a double dose of a harmful gene. It appears that's what had happened in this case.

Farooqi, who had only recently joined the lab, ran a blood test for leptin on both children, not thinking she would reveal anything other than the high level she expected. Instead she found nothing. Not even a hint of leptin. Thinking she must have done the tests wrong, she ran them again. Still nothing. The team had found the first human carriers of the ob gene.

These children were getting fatter because, without leptin, their bodies were telling their brains that they were starving, prompting insatiable hunger. Hunger is a very primal drive, like thirst or sleep. Although we understand the drive to sleep, we find it much more difficult to understand the concept of someone who cannot stop eating. We assume that they must be able to control themselves and that what we are seeing can only be extreme gluttony, which revolts many people. But people with defective ob genes have absolutely no control over their appetite – you might as well tell them to stop breathing.

Injections of leptin seemed an obvious solution, but it had never been used on children before and it took months of agonizing before all the ethical approval hurdles had been cleared. Once on leptin the children rapidly lost both weight and their appetite. Both had also had little resistance to infection and abnormally low levels of reproductive hormones. Without treatment, neither child would have gone through puberty. With leptin treatment, the older child has already developed normally.

What's evident from this story is that genes can have a major influence on body size. Twin studies show that between 40 and 70 per cent of fat mass is heritable. We know this instinctively. Tall thin people beget more like them. Short round people have short round children. Despite this evidence all around us, we persist in thinking that fat is simply about self-indulgent behaviour. Of course genes have not altered much in the last fifty years and blame for the explosion in obesity cannot be laid solely at their door. Lack of exercise and change in diet have been key to the rise in obesity. This doesn't alter the fact that whether we put on fat quickly or slowly is also due to the gene combinations we get dealt at conception.

When, in 2004, the House of Commons Health Select Committee issued a report on obesity, they chose, in the second paragraph of the report, to highlight the case of a grossly obese child who had died aged three, 'choked by her fat', as an example of Britain's fat future. Most parents of three year olds will tell you that getting them to eat is far more difficult than stopping them eating, and somehow this story of a chip-chomping, couch-potato toddler didn't ring true. When it was revealed that this child too came from the Bengali community, I thought immediately of the cousins treated in Cambridge. The unit confirmed that the chances of a three-year-old child being this obese without having underlying disease was vanishingly small.

'Fat and dead . . . at 3' was the headline in *The Sun*. 'Shock at tot killed by weight problem' it continued. The tenor of this piece and several others was that the parents were to blame. Clearly they must have been feeding the child a diet of pizza, chips and crisps. There were some deeply unpleasant comments in the media which revealed the true loathing of fat, with a constant implication throughout that it was purely about self-indulgence. Letters in the *Daily Mail* said the parents were unfit to raise children, and called for them to be taken away.

Appalled, I ran a piece in *The Guardian*, pointing out that the parents of a child with any other genetic disease would not be pilloried in this way, and the child could no more help being fat than one with cystic fibrosis could help having lung problems. At this point, the Cambridge unit announced that they had been treating the child, who did indeed have a genetic disease affecting her hormones, and it was then the turn of the Select Committee chairman to feel uncomfortable. Perhaps the commentators too felt sheepish about jumping to conclusions so readily, for their subsequent attack on the Committee chairman was ferocious. Many Britons would benefit from the cycle lanes and much-reduced fat intake trumpeted as obesity solutions in the Committee's report. To suggest that those with hormone defects could be cured by the same measures is wilfully cruel. Yet this is what other doctors at the hospital treating this child were quoted as saying, in a report published in the *Daily Mail*.

Dr Nigel Meadows, a consultant paediatrician at the same hospital, said of the three-year-old: 'It was a shocking case. You don't imagine your kid is just going to die of **obesity**. The parents were devastated. Some may say the parents are responsible, but if a child is demanding food it can be very difficult to refuse it.'

The doctors made four key observations to the committee: that prevention was the only solution; that the availability of food high in fat and sugar must be reduced; that exercise must be reintroduced into school curricula; and that education about healthy eating must be compulsory for all school children.

Not one of these recommendations would have made any difference to that particular child.

So an aberration in the gene that carries the instructions for producing the hormone leptin can result in gross obesity. The actual hormone is only part of leptin's pathway to the control centre – it won't work without its receptors. Defective instructions for the leptin receptor can also cause less severe early-onset obesity, as can faults in other receptors within the control centre of the fat thermostat, the hypothalamus. One gene of particular interest is for a type of receptor called MC4R. It picks up incoming signals from a protein activated by leptin and then relays a message that says 'I'm full, stop eating.' O'Rahilly's team can look at the DNA sequence for this gene in the very obese and then predict – very accurately – how much they will eat for breakfast. More aberrations in the sequence means more food. A completely non-functioning MC4R and you'll eat three times as much breakfast as people without this mutation.

Some of us are born to binge. There is a strong link between mutations in a gene involved in the leptin hormone pathway and binge-eating. All twenty-four severely obese people in a study reported in the *New England Journal of Medicine*, 2003, who had an MC4R mutation were binge-eaters, while only 14 per cent of 445 other obese patients were bingers.

Mutations of MC4R are the commonest found in the leptin hormone pathway, accounting for one in twenty of those severely obese seen by the Cambridge team. There's a curious footnote to this: people with this mutation also tend to have red hair and pale skin.

Whereas the prominent absence of leptin is the trigger for gross obesity, it is usual for those who are fat to have lots of leptin – in fact the amount they have is proportional to their fat mass. The body's response on hearing lots of leptin noise should be to throttle back the eating and up energy expenditure, but in the obese the hypothalamus is deaf to leptin's messages, no matter how many of them there are. The body has become leptin-resistant. Thus the appropriate obesity response – eat less, expend more energy – is not forthcoming. While leptin gene aberrations are very rare, leptin resistance is probably rather common. If your fat thermostat has been reset, more and more leptin is produced (in just the same way that more insulin is produced in Type 2 diabetes) only to produce a less than optimal response.

So leptin, then, is the hormone that signals how fat you are, whose job is to maintain fat stores at a constant level. If there is no signal from leptin, the fat controller in the hypothalamus assumes that there is no fat and initiates desperate measures to up fat levels. It's an example of a negative-feedback loop. In many ways, leptin is rather an unusual hormone. In fact, it works a bit like a vitamin. You have to have some, but having significantly more doesn't seem to make any difference.

Leptin does, however, have a long-term strategic role in regulating our lives. We have already seen in Chapter 3 that it is a key player in puberty. When the percentage of body fat reaches a certain threshold level, it is messages from leptin that persuade the hypothalamus and pituitary between them to initiate puberty. Equally, when messages are no longer being received – because body fat drops so low in the dangerously lean, such as ballet dancers, athletes and anorexics – reproduction is switched off. Some elegant work at the Harvard Medical School by Professor Christo Mantzoros showed that injecting leptin into women athletes who had had, on average, no periods for five years, restored menstruation, seemingly by getting luteinising hormone to be released in pulses once more. It's a system that has developed to protect not us, but our potential offspring, from a less than optimal start in life.

The Hormone of Hunger – Ghrelin

The discovery of leptin has prompted a gold rush of further hormone discovery around appetite. For instance, how does your body know when to stop eating because you are full up? An obvious mechanism is via nerves that run from the gut to the brain which are fired by physical distension of the gut – that too-stuffed-to-move feeling. The problem with this theory, although there are nerves that undoubtedly do this, is that a meal of boiled cabbage can still leave you feeling hungry, even though you feel completely bloated. Nor does putting 600 calories in through a line intra-venously make you feel full the way that a 600-calorie Big Mac does.

Let me present *ghrelin* (usually pronounced 'grellin' but you may also hear 'graylin'), the hormone of hunger, which is produced by the stomach – and its kissing cousin, *PYY*, the hormone of satiety (feeling full), produced by the intestine.

Hormone doctors and researchers are dazzled by ghrelin. At the recent World Congress of Endocrinology in Lisbon, every session on ghrelin was packed to the rafters. It's a tiny chain of amino acids, produced by single cells in the stomach and a fantastically potent appetite-booster or as, scientists would say, an orexigen (which is a great Scrabble word). Inject ghrelin and suddenly you are not just peckish, but could eat a horse. Ghrelin levels fall when you have just had a meal and are at their highest during fasting.

Steve Bloom is head of the Division of Investigative Science at Imperial College; he and his team work at the Hammersmith Hospital. Researchers at the Hammersmith gave injections of either ghrelin or saline to volunteers and found that those who had had the hormone infusion ate 30 per cent more.

There seems to be a food pecking order with ghrelin. Levels fall most in response to carbohydrate, then protein, and finally fat, which is interesting because it could be one reason why we are seeing a rise in obesity with modern diets. During the Second World War, for instance, the diet was high in carbohydrates like potatoes and bread but low in fats, and hunger was fully sated by that diet. Today we get more of our calories from fats, which don't provoke such a large fall in ghrelin, so you are still hungry despite a big meal.

Circulating ghrelin is increased in those people on low-calorie diets, those with cancer, anorexia and other wasting diseases. If you lose weight because you've dieted, ghrelin levels respond in a compensatory way, making you hungrier so you'll put that lost weight back on again – a classic case of hormones working against you. Interestingly, however, weight loss following low-fat diets does not trigger a ghrelin adjustment, suggesting why these diets are more effective long-term ways to lose weight.

In June 2004, researchers from the University of California at Los Angeles (UCLA), led by Dr Julio Licinio, discovered that in lean men's blood there is a giant burst of ghrelin between midnight and 6 a.m., which exceeds normal pre-mealtime surges. There was no such peak in obese men, suggesting that obesity itself down-regulates ghrelin. It defies the image of a fat man raiding the fridge at night, driven by insatiable hunger. Much of this new work redefines the popular notion of fat people's behaviour.

The Hormone that Says 'I'm Full Up' – PYY

PYY (or PYY_{3-36} to be strictly accurate) is the exact opposite to ghrelin, in that it is low in fasting and rises after a meal. It inhibits appetite, and if you give this one to volunteers, they eat 30 per cent *less* food. What is particularly interesting is that they stay less hungry the next day too. The more calories you eat, the bigger the rise in PYY. This is why the huge calorie intake that is a Sunday roast with all the trimmings, plus pudding, results in you being not that hungry at breakfast on Monday. Slowly digested foods like high-fibre ones, give an even bigger rise, which is why you continue to feel full for longer if you choose to eat wholemeal pasta, for instance, rather than the normal variety. Again, comparing us to our grandparents, perhaps refined foods don't cause such a big rise in PYY, so we go on eating. Neither of these hormones seems to have any other side effects.

The control of appetite is both hormonal and neural. These two hormones – ghrelin and PYY – both act on the hypothalamus, which has two responses – eat more and eat less – both mediated through neurotransmitters. The eat-less part works via the MC4R receptor that we mentioned earlier. The eat-more ones are called NPY (neuropeptide Y) and AgRP. Both are inhibited by leptin, but it is ghrelin that switches on the neurons that make you eat and switches off the ones that dampen your appetite. PYY does exactly the opposite.

I know I am a hormone enthusiast, and probably far too easily pleased, but as an example of hormones at their most elegant, this system takes some beating. So very clever when it works – but so awful when it doesn't.

Thin Drugs, Fat Profits

So, at one extreme, we have genetically determined problems with hormones or their pathways as a cause of gross obesity, mostly commencing in childhood. Then there is the middle ground as it were, where the response of our hormones to the things that we do (or don't do), like exercise and overeat, makes us fat – and sometimes very, very fat. There are relatively small numbers of people in the first category – possibly 5 per cent of those who are obese – but the numbers in the second category run to tens of millions. Knowing this has drug companies rubbing their hands in glee. For if hormones make you fat, can they not also be used to make you thin?

In 1893 thyroid extracts began to be marketed for weight loss under brand names like 'Safe Fat Reducer' and 'Corpulin'. As you now know, thyroid extract is the one hormone that can safely navigate the gut, but safe it ain't. Given in excess it can cause sudden death, not to mention bone loss, palpitations and weakness, as muscles are burned up in its all-consuming quest for fuel to increase metabolism. In order to avoid these alarming side effects, patients were advised to take 'chasers' of arsenic or even strychnine.

Hormones were not the only diet fixes. Laxatives too were very popular as was a particularly nasty chemical called dinitrophenol, a diet aid of the 1920s. An ingredient of explosives and weed killers, it too had a nasty habit of killing people. The idea of increasing metabolism persisted, however, and in the 1940s, digitalis, better known as a heart medication, was introduced as a treatment for weight loss. Amphetamines were touted for the same purpose at around the same time and were prescribed indiscriminately to two thirds of those seeking advice on weight control. Their side effects – psychiatric disorders, addiction, withdrawal problems, heart failure, sudden death – were well known but largely swept under the carpet. It wasn't a lesson learned. Fenfluramine and phentermine, both licensed individually for dieters in the 1970s by the FDA, began to be used together and by 1996, despite media scares, 18 million prescriptions a year were issued for illegal 'off label' (i.e. not for indications licensed by regulators) use of what came to be known as fen-phen. It caused long lingering deaths from primary pulmonary hypertension and valvular heart disease. By the late 1990s, fen and phen and another similar drug, dexfenfluramine, had finally disappeared.

This illustrates two things: first, the intense desire for such products by the overweight, even with knowledge of their potential side effects; and second, nothing that is both really effective and relatively free of side effects has yet been invented, even though a fortune awaits its inventors.

A successful obesity drug is top of every drug company's wish list. At the time of writing, there are two, neither of which are particularly effective (weight loss with proper use of around 5 per cent), and both have side effects. The drug orlistat (Xenical) attempts to stop food being absorbed by altering the action of a fat-busting enzyme, which prevents fats from being broken down and thus absorbed. About a third of dietary fat exits via the stools. If you don't cut down the level of fat in your diet whilst taking Xenical, you get what the company euphemistically calls 'anal leakage'. Nice. Sibutramine (Reductil) works in a different way in that it affects neurotransmitters in the brain involved in appetite. One of its side effects is an increase in blood pressure, the very last thing you want in the seriously obese, who usually already have blood pressure problems.

So why don't the companies just target the neurotransmitters involved in switching off appetite – by developing an anti-NPY molecule, for example? The problem here is that this neurotransmitter is found all over the brain and does far more than just regulate appetite. Thus the likelihood of an anti-NPY drug causing side effects is very high and on this rocky shore have foundered many attempts which target the brain circuits controlling appetite. Of 114 anti-fat products that began development, just four have made it all the way through to clinical trials.

The discovery of leptin has led to an explosion of new hormonal discovery and a plethora of potential new anti-fat targets for the pharmaceutical companies. For instance, oxyntomodulin is a newly discovered pre-hormone, which inhibits appetite and is released in the gut in proportion to meal size. It is found in high quantities in those conditions associated with low bodyweight, such as anorexia. But knowing what these things do and understanding how to develop them as effective drugs are very different. An example would be giving people PYY so that they would constantly feel too full to eat much. The problem here is that PYY is a peptide, which means that it would be destroyed by the gut if taken orally, so would have to be injected – and on a daily basis to be effective. Daily injections are just not practical for the purposes of mass medication.

Ghrelin is proving to be a shining star, endocrinologically speaking. It's been discovered that it is what's called a secretagogue for growth hormone – triggering its production. Far from just acting in the stomach and in the brain, ghrelin receptors have been found in the heart, pancreas, testis and placenta. What on earth is it doing there?

One of the best ways to find out what something does in the body is to breed mice engineered *not* to have the gene that makes whatever it is that you are interested in. These are called knockout mice. From all you've heard so far, you'd think ghrelin-deficient mice would be teeny and ever so skinny. Actually they're not, they're of normal size and weight but interestingly they do seem to have cardiovascular problems as they age. This suggests ghrelin might have a role in maintaining metabolism during ageing. Ghrelin also seems to be implicated in sleep and in the regulation of anxiety. Truth to tell, there's decades of research left in ghrelin. If there was one hormone in this book that I would tip as the one to watch, it's this one. I suspect that you may possibly see the first use of ghrelin, not in the obese but as a weight controller in cancer patients who have lost too much weight.

The Hormone of Energy Balance — Adiponectin

The discovery of leptin, a hormone produced by the most unlikely of endocrine organs, fat, prompted researchers to look again at our blubbery stuff, and in 2001 it was announced that another hormone had been found. *Adiponectin* has a role in regulating energy balance, seemingly raising metabolic rate. Its production is not distributed evenly across our fat, but concentrated in our love handles and other unsavoury bulgy bits that migrate to our middles. Unlike leptin, where high levels are linked with being overweight, there's a negative association between adiponectin and obesity. Low circulating levels of adiponectin have now been discovered to be a very accurate pre-dictor of Type 2 diabetes risk. The lower the adiponectin, the worse the blood fats profile, the greater the risk of heart disease being asso-ciated with the diabetes.

The threads of this story are now beginning to come together. At the beginning, we talked about insulin, the hormone which controls sugar levels in the body by telling cells all over the body, in the liver and muscle, to absorb glucose from the blood. When people get Type 2 diabetes, first their muscles and liver, but not their fat, become insulin-resistant, meaning that despite production of increasing amounts of insulin, their cells are deaf to its exhortation to take up glucose. Too much fat, as we know, is likely to cause

Type 2 diabetes – but curiously having too little causes exactly the same disease.

People who have a disease called lipodystrophy have almost no fat. You can have such a condition from birth, or acquire it because of something like HIV. It sounds vaguely attractive, but actually is very disfiguring, making people look permanently sick and skeletal. Because the bodies of those with lipodystrophy can't store fat, their bodies try to move it into muscle tissue or the liver instead. In people who are obese, there is also nowhere to store fat, but in their case it's not because there is no fat, but because all the fat depots are already full to brimming. Just as in those with no fat, there is an attempt to shift it to muscle and liver. In both the obese and the thin, the consequence, especially in muscle, is that fatty acids spill into the cells, somehow altering the normal response to insulin. It is possible that adiponectin is the missing link between insulin resistance and obesity. If it is, it means that diabetes is not the sugar problem we've thought it was for the best part of eighty-five years, but a fat problem. As I write, no adiponectin is yet available for use in humans. When it can be made in sufficient quantity for human use, as it surely will, we may discover that this hormone can be used for treating both obesity and diabetes. But so far this is just surmise.

When I tell people that hormones can make them fat and about the fat thermostat, there are two reactions. One is relief and the other is suspicion, usually followed by 'But it's still about putting too much in and not enough out', which for the majority of people is right. For years, management of obesity has been about the management of behaviour. I hope that this chapter has persuaded you that behaviour is only part of the obesity problem. The other part is hormones. And that's the truth.

CHAPTER EIGHT

HORMONES AS CLOCKS

Although we sometimes lose track of time and are surprised to discover the hour, our bodies have usually already reminded us that it's way past bedtime, or that we should have eaten lunch an hour ago. Actually, our bodies are very good at keeping time and can count not just in minutes or months but in years too. The biological clocks we have on board help keep our bodies running on schedule, because we are complicated machines and our efficient running depends not on pell-mell, anything-goes activity, but on a carefully timetabled programme. Hormones, for example, are not released any old how, but in a carefully controlled way. Growth hormone at night, testosterone in the early morning, gonadotrophin releasing hormone every ninety minutes and so on.

Although we may think that we are agents of free will, much of what we do, and more pertinently, when we do it, is dictated by our body clock. Here again we find hormones in the thick of it. Not only is the messenger slave of the body clock a hormone, melatonin, but many of our other hormones can also have a time-warping effect, making time appear to run either more quickly or more slowly. The truth about hormones and time is the subject of this chapter.

Hormones and Stopwatches

If something interests you – reading this chapter, for instance – time will seem to pass quickly. But if – and I hope this is unlikely – you are already bored by the end of this paragraph, time will appear to drag. This effect – think of it as the 'watched kettle' syndrome – is not just an artefact of our mind but the hallmark of a 'stopwatch' in the brain, the so-called interval timer that marks spans of up to two hours. The onset of an event lasting a familiar amount of time – say a traffic light at the bottom of your road changing to red – activates the start button of the interval timer which is located in the brain. Hitting 'start' gets a particular sub-set of nerves that normally fire at will to sing from the same songsheet, as it were, and to fire in a coordinated way. Meanwhile, a whoosh of the nerve transmitter dopamine is released. Both of these things together wake up a particular set of brain cells, which proceed to monitor this unusual phenomenon until the nerves return to their random pattern of yore.

So, your red-light watching creates a unique pattern and when, once again, you are sitting in front of that light, and the pattern begins once more, the monitor in the brain (actually spiny cells in the striatum, if you want the science) recognizes and tracks it. When the monitor reckons (from past experience) the red light should turn to amber, it sends a 'time's up' signal to the decision-making centres of the brain. For people with diseases that affect dopamine release – like Parkinson's – time runs slow, and they consistently underesti-mate the length of intervals of time. Marijuana has the same effect. On the other hand, recreational stimulants like cocaine and amphet-amine, which increase the availability of dopamine, expand time. Stress hormones, such as cortisol or adrenaline, can also slow down the sense of time passing as they too increase dopamine. This is why, during stressful, nasty experiences, every second feels like an hour. It's also why, when you are late, and freaked out by traffic, with your child still waiting on the school's doorstep to be collected, red lights cruelly seem to stay red for ever. It's your hormones tinkering with your interval timer.

Down Memory Lane with Your Hormones

Now let me digress a moment, to think about times past. Many people are able to recall where they were when they heard a particular piece of news – 9/11 for instance, or the assassination of President Kennedy. Here, the emotions of an event that we perceive to be highly consequential to our lives seem to burnish memory. It is very clear that stress hormones affect memory formation, as memories recorded at the time of a traumatic or very emotional event appear to be 'burnt in', remaining vivid for decades. There is an odd flashbulb effect to these memories, with some aspects (not always the most important) being recorded in minute detail, while others are hazy. For instance, someone might remember a brooch on a dress of woman involved in an accident, but not the style or length of the dress or what she was carrying, or another detail altogether – the noise made by rain falling, or a smell – yet not who was standing next to them at the time.

One of the most miserable days of my life took place on a quiet sunny day in September 1997. For fifteen years, I ran a mother and baby research charity, and for twelve of them worked closely with Diana, the Princess of Wales, who was the charity's patron. She was not only very dear to me, but had been a hugely important part of my working life. As I stood in Westminster Abbey, waiting for the arrival of the coffin, I was struggling to stay in control. Then, amid unbearable silence, came a creak, creak sound. It was the noise made by the boots of the guardsmen bearing the coffin. I remember every moment of the next hour and the way, as the coffin left, that overwhelming grief forced its way from somewhere visceral to emerge in a choking soundless howl. To this day I have no idea of who was next to me or how I got home. About two months later I was making a programme on hypnosis for the BBC. I did not considered myself suggestible, but the hypnotist Paul McKenna still managed to hypnotize me. The producers told me that I had sat there for twenty-five minutes with tears rolling down my face. When Paul asked me what I had been thinking of, the words simply fell out of my mouth unbidden. The creak of the guardsmen's boots. Such is the power of memory burnt into the brain's circuits by hormones.

The hippocampus, which plays a critical role in memory tasks and spatial learning, is the area of the brain which is richest in stress hormone receptors. Sudden acute elevations of the stress hormone cortisol enhance memory formation, while chronic long-term exposure can cause black holes in the memory. Typically memory is a problem for those with depression, in whom cortisol levels are elevated.

Why should such memory-enhancing occur? With traumatic events, it is about survival. The stress hormone rush that accompanies a near-death moment and the subsequent laying down of memory ensures that you learn from it, and don't make the same mistake twice. Unfortunately for those with post traumatic stress disorder, this survival tactic has become so overwhelming as to be severely disabling, with vivid memories being a constant intrusion.

The Hormone of Sleep and Time — Melatonin

The circadian clock (from *circa* – about, and *diem* – a day) tunes our bodies to the cycles of light and dark caused by the earth's rotation. The clock synchronizes our activity so that we are at our most active when food, sunlight and prey are available (or, in our modern age, when Sainsbury's is open). It also prioritizes certain types of behaviour with the seasons – nesting in spring, hibernating in autumn – which ensures that young are produced when food is at its most plentiful.

The clock doesn't just control cycles of sleep and wakefulness but also rigorously schedules our physiology. Under its influence, the activity of almost every system in the body varies predictably across a twenty-four-hour period. For instance, our body temperature peaks in the early evening (as those of you with fretful children with fevers will know) and drops to its nadir at about 4.30 in the morning, as does concentration and cognitive processing. Urine collection is suppressed overnight, with bowel movements similarly hobbled from about about 10.30 p.m. The most likely time for your bowel to evacuate the remains of yesterday's lunch and supper is 8.30 a.m. Blood pressure rises very sharply at about 6.45 a.m., reaching a peak at 6.30 p.m. You are at your perkiest and most alert at 10 a.m., with best coordination at 2.30 p.m. Maximal sports performance is in the early evening – which is when most world records are broken – perhaps not surprising since this time is when cardiovascular efficiency, muscle strength and flexibility are all at their daily peak.

Hormones, too, are under the clock's domain. For instance, twenty times as much cortisol is produced in the morning (between 4 and 8 a.m.), growth hormone and prolactin, the hormone of milk production, are secreted in greatest quantity an hour after sleep, and testosterone drives libido hardest, as it were, first thing in the morning. It's not just daily rhythm of hormone production that is set by the clock. Hormones change with the seasons, in animals at least, and with passing time, from puberty, when the hormones that prompt action within testis and ovary are pumped out, mostly at night, in industrial quantities, to adulthood, when these are secreted in pulsed doses throughout a twenty-four-hour period.

The clock is set by light, which is just as well, because away from light the clock lacks the precision we expect of the finest timepieces. Tucked deep in a cave, our true rhythms would show themselves – and although they are close to twenty-four hours, they're consistently out – 24.2-hour days to be exact, or, for some blind people, twenty-five hour days. So what, you might say, an extra twelve minutes a day – does it matter? Actually it matters a great deal. Over a period of time we would drift out of phase with the sun, and do inappropriate things, like (if we were mice) emerge from burrows at inadvisable times, or (as humans), sleep through Sunday lunch or want to shop at 3 a.m. Every day, the clock is reset through our exposure to light, and has a preference for natural light. We think, particularly in the dead of winter, that it is brighter inside than outside. Actually, we are deceived: soon after dawn, natural light is fifty times brighter than normal office lighting. At noon, natural light is up to a thousand times brighter. Even in winter. Even in Britain.

So where is this clock and how does it work? Is there a hormone in it somewhere? You bet.

Ten years ago, little was known about biological clocks. Today clock-watching is a major theme in biology and biological 'clocks' have been found everywhere, even in the simplest organisms, like blue-green algae. All our tissues also seem to have their own little clocks, which beat to a drum-beat set by the master clock, which in mammals is located in the suprachiasmatic nucleus (SCN). The brain tracks fluctuations in light with the help of cells in the retina, at the back of the eye. A pigment in the cells detects light and sends information about its brightness and duration to the SCN, which dispatches information to all the bits of the brain that control daily rhythms, including, via a relay station, the pineal gland, which secretes the hormone melatonin.

Now let me introduce you properly to the pineal gland, known to the ancients as the third eye. A little dangle of glandular tissue protruding from the mid-brain, somewhere behind the eyes, it was known primarily as a photo receptor in animals like frogs and salamanders. If you're thinking, how could it detect light inside the skull, remember back to when you were a child and reading under the bedclothes with a torch. Putting a hand over the torch still lets light through. This is certainly the case in amphibian and reptile skulls, although not in human skulls.

This titchy gland has always provoked heated debate, not least amongst physiologists. Some were convinced that it had an important role in sexual activities and reproduction, while other physiologists claimed it was nothing but sexual delusion on their part. In

1954 a review of pineal tumours in humans showed that those that destroyed the pineal were associated with advanced sexual development while those that originated from it were linked to delayed sexual development. By 1958, the pineal hormone had been isolated. It was called melatonin, because in amphibians this hormone moves the granules that contain melanin (the pigment of moles and freckles) to the centre of the cell thereby lightening the skin. It is also related as well as to the brain transmitter serotonin. By 1973, it had been noted that the levels of melatonin in the blood varied and that although scarcely detectable during the day, they soared during the hours of darkness. Now we know that melatonin is not only the hormone of sleep, but also the hormone slave of the body clock – relentlessly coordinating our activity so that it is in step with our environment, night or day, summer or winter, spring or fall.

The pineal is an unusual gland, in that it is like the middle bit of the adrenal gland, the part that secretes fight or flight adrenaline, producing its hormone not in response to something circulating in the blood, but rather in response to nervous stimulation. The suprachiasmatic nucleus (SCN) receives information from cells at the back of the eye. The SCN tells the pineal when it is daytime, not by a direct signal but by sending a message to another brain region, the paraventricular nucleus. The effect of SCN's message is to stop it telling the pineal gland to release melatonin. After dark, the SCN releases the brake, allowing the paraventricular nucleus to carry on relaying its 'secrete melatonin now' message.

If mammals lose their eyes, they are both visually blind and circadian blind, having no synchronisation of their twenty-four-hour patterns to the light dark cycle. If birds, reptiles of fish lose their eyes, they are blind but still maintain synchronisation of their daily rhythms because they have several light-sensing receptors elsewhere in their bodies. So there was huge excitement when it was suggested that humans might also have light receptors elsewhere – in the back of their knees.

In 1998, Scott Campbell and Pat Murphy of Cornell University

Medical College in White Plains, New York, published research in *Science* showing that shining strong light on the backs of a person's knees could reset their body clock. To say that this was a bombshell was an understatement. It opened up the prospect that, perhaps, as groggy shiftworkers, January depressives and jet-lagged executives slept, they could be treated with blasts of light aimed kneewards. Excitement turned to dismay as group after group of researchers failed to replicate the experiment. Finally, in 2002, the idea was firmly nailed following work from Harvard. Only light reaching the eyes can reset the clock. All a torch behind your knees will do is warm the skin.

Here's a peculiarity. It was assumed that rods and cones, which are the specialized cells of vision that sit at the back of the eye, must be crucial to clock-setting. In mice that lack rods and cones in their eyes there is still a synchroised circardian rhythm. In humans too, some of those people who are blind through loss of sight may still have a synchronised circadian rhythm, while those who are blind because they have no eyes, do not, which has always been a puzzle. It seems that at the back of the eye there's a tangle of nerves, a bit like the tangle of wire behind the back of the TV, and here, there are photo-receptors, which contain a pigment called melanopsin, which reacts to light in the blue part of the spectrum. For humans, light at the blue end of the spectrum is twice as biologically effective in setting our clock as any other sort.

The strong effect of light on our biological clock presents many problems for night-shift workers. Even after twenty years of night shifts, individuals will still not have shifted their circadian rhythm in response to the demands of working at night. That's a big problem because night-shift workers do many important jobs in which safety is critical – from cab drivers to doctors to power station workers. All of them will experience that same dip of concentration and body temperature that the rest of us do around 4–5 am. Taking account of the amount of traffic on the roads, the risk of a road traffic accident occurring at 6 a.m. is twenty times that at 10 a.m. It is no coincidence that 6 a.m. is just when night-shift workers are going home. It is also noticeable that many of the major industrial accidents occur at night: Three Mile Island at 4 a.m., Union Carbide plant, Bhopal, at 12.15 a.m., and Chernobyl at 1.23 a.m.

There also appears to be a significant effect on health of night-shift working. For instance, there is an increased cardiovascular mortality compared to the normal population, higher rates of substance abuse, difficulty in sleeping, greater levels of depression, and also, significantly, more infertility, particularly in women. This is not surprising. Reproductive processes in animals must be closely matched to the environment's clock, or else young would be produced at the wrong time. Disruption of the pineal or of the clock genes causes disruption of the reproductive cycles and mid-pregnancy loss in mice. Tumours affecting the pineal gland in human advance or delay puberty and play havoc with fertility. Although we might like to think of ourselves as non-seasonal animals, there is in fact a sharp jump in births in spring, which indicates that seasonality has not been entirely wiped from our systems. This effect is even more marked in the Scandinavian countries. Although there may be a seasonal variation in sexual activity – summer holidays leading to spring-time births – the fact that there is a direct effect on fertility is shown by seasonal variations in the quality of embryos and fertilization rates in women undergoing IVF procedures.

There are some interesting studies of female flight attendants, who show increased rates of breast cancer, that are greater than would be expected simply from the extra exposure to radiation that flight crews experience. It is put down to disruption of circadian rhythm. We'll come to using circadian rhythm for treatment in a moment.

So why don't night-shift workers adjust in the same way that we adjust to local time when we travel across multiple time zones? Their problem is that they have to go home. And in doing so, almost invariably, they are exposed to natural light while travelling, which as we've said, even shortly after dawn, is very bright. Thus their clocks are reset. As a result, night-workers show an abnormal phasing of their melatonin rhythm. Levels are often high when they are awake (but should be asleep) and low when they are trying to rest.

Timed light is the obvious treatment for jet lag but that presents many practical difficulties, which is why melatonin is the treatment of choice for many. It can be bought over the counter in any drugstore in the US, where, astonishingly, it is classified as a food supplement.

Today we live in a 24/7 society. My local supermarket is open twenty-four hours a day, and if I wanted to I could play all night on e-Bay, or go out clubbing until dawn. Our parents couldn't do any of these things, because shops shut at 6 p.m, or much earlier if you lived outside London. So potentially we can live life constantly exposed to light, when in theory it should be dark. Our bodies are pretty confused by this degree of light pollution and it has been suggested that inappropriate light signals may be affecting our sleep patterns.

All animals sleep. Birds do it, bees do it and yes, pretty certainly, educated fleas do it too. Certainly Drosophila, those tiny flies that cluster around rotting fruit, do. Fish too. Dolphins slumber with one half of their brain awake and the other half asleep. We all need to sleep, for without sleep, we sicken and die remarkably quickly. In fact, almost as quickly as if we had been deprived of water. Sleep is one of the great enigmas of science, because although clearly physical recovery is an important aspect of it – both for body and mind – there's far more to it than that. There are four stages of sleep, with the body cycling between two quite different types: REM (rapid eye movement) sleep, and a deep sleep in which we are both blind and paralysed. Each has a different function – but what? There are many theories: consolidation of memory is one, switching the brain 'offline' for repairs is another. But it could be several of these things – or quite possibly none of them.

Over each twenty-four-hour period, we are pushed and pulled by two opposing forces. Our circadian rhythm pushes us to be alert during day. There is also a strong biological drive for sleep, which increases the longer you have been awake. By 10 p.m., we are still surprisingly perky, despite having had many hours without sleep. This is the circadian wakefulness drive at work. When we do sleep, we have probably satisfied our sleep debt by about 4 a.m., yet we tend to sleep on for a few hours – that's the other bit of the push-me pull-you. We see the true extent of the battle between these opposing forces in people who are allowed to sleep one hour in every three over several days, and yet, despite severe sleep deprivation, are still unable to sleep during afternoon and early evening peaks of the circadian cycle. A win on points for our circadian rhythms?

The duration of sleep is very accurately regulated and it becomes increasingly easy to wake in the morning with age. We tend to be either larks or owls, something that is genetically determined. If your mother drives you mad by getting up at 5 a.m., chances are that you are going there too as you age.

Early to bed and early to rise, makes a man healthy, wealthy and wise is something our parents have all parroted at us. Benjamin Franklin said it first and he was wrong. A 1998 research study from two researchers at Southampton University showed no association between getting up and going to bed early and health, socio-economic or cognitive advantage. If anything, owls were wealthier than larks.

About 3 per cent of people in the UK suffer from seasonal affective disorder (SAD). They become depressed as winter draws on, cutting down their activity. They crave carbohydrates and often put on lots of weight, only beginning to feel better in the spring, when they become active again. Since melatonin release is suppressed by light, the onset of shorter days means fewer hours of daylight so that the blood is carrying more melatonin than it would in summer when the days are long. It is said that SAD is a leftover of our past, the way that cavemen became semi-hibernating creatures during the winter months. The problem seems to be that while healthy people can take light cues from artificial light as well as from natural light, those with SAD respond only to the natural form. Carefully timed bright light in the blue spectrum can be a very successful treatment.

There's an element here of another effect of melatonin – energy balance. Melatonin is a key factor in seasonal behaviours, like hibernation. One of the things that animals do before they hibernate is tuck away fat stores and then, during hibernation, their metabolism slows to a crawl. Melatonin will have an influence on humans too. You may well have found your excuse for the accumulation of post-Christmas blubber: my melatonin made me do it.

Jet lag is a phenomenon of our age. When your internal clock is telling a different time to that of your wristwatch, your body is in deep confusion. It can take anything up to a week to recover and you tend to feel worse, not the day after, but the one after that. Mental alertness disappears, your stomach is somewhere in California still and you don't know what time of day it is. Jet lag's effects are far more noticeable flying from west to east, than the other way around, so much so that analysis of the records of American West coast baseball teams playing away games on the East coast showed that the home team consistently scored more runs when their opponents had just flown across time zones for the match. Why should travelling west to east be worse? East to west means going with your clock's flow. By inclination, it wants longer days. Going in the other direction means a transitional period of shorter days.

Taking melatonin can prevent jet lag, but it doesn't work for everybody and it must be taken by your destination's clock to be successful. It is not worth using for time zone changes of less than five hours. If travelling west, you need to delay the onset of sleep, so you should take a dose of melatonin (about 5 mg) at your destination's bedtime (say 11 p.m.) for four nights. If travelling east, you need to advance the onset of sleep. Take a pill on the flight when it would be your destination's bedtime. When you arrive, take a dose at the destination bedtime for four nights. Melatonin is not available in Europe except on prescription.

Melatonin is also very useful in treating the sleep problems of the blind: nearly 60 per cent report problems with sleeping and this proportion increases with increasing degree of loss of light perception.

Body Rhythms as Medicine

Using the body's rhythms to help in treatment – so-called chronotherapeutics – is not that new an idea, but it is one that has still to take off. For instance, the risk of relapse in children with acute lymphoblastic leukaemia is two and a half times higher in children who receive their chemotherapy in the morning than those having the same treatment in the evening. This is because genes that regulate cell proliferation (in other words, the ones that are especially active in cancers) are under clock control. Disruption of the clock genes seems to accelerate tumour growth in rats, so it is not surprising perhaps that night-shift workers show an increase in cancer rates.

Melatonin – hormone of darkness and slave to the body clock – coordinates physiology on a grand scale, as we can see, not only through the day and night but through the seasons too. By affecting the release of other hormones, it also influences mood, reproduction and energy balance. It has a powerful anti-oxidant effect, which could be why low levels are associated with cancers. Since levels fall with age, you may already have guessed that melatonin is one of the most popular of all hormones with the rejuvenators *de nos jours*. In the next chapter, I'll tell you how immortality is but a hormone away.

CHAPTER NINE

HOLDING BACK THE YEARS

In 2005 – just as in 1905, when the word hormone was first coined – there are two hormone 'tracks'. Science-based endocrinology is one road, while the other is extravagant quackery, which, on the face of it, is making pretty much the same claims as were made a hundred years ago. The logic of today's breed of rejuvenators is not dissimilar to that of Brown-Séquard, the pioneer of hormones, who ended an otherwise distinguished career by trying to restore that which was lost, by injections of semen. The gist of the rejuvenators' argument is this: since the levels of many hormones are known to fall with age, restoring hormone levels to those of youth will hold back the years. The truth about hormones is not quite that obvious.

Trying to regain youth is a pursuit that is millennia old. The Bible tells us, rather indiscreetly, that King David had a significant loss of 'heat' as he reached his twilight years. A solution was found in the form of Abishag (surely a case of nominative determinism if ever there was one), a virgin from the Shunammite tribe. 'Let her lie in thy bosom that my lord the king may get heat,' said his counsellors, who possibly were hoping for the idea to catch on so that they too could have a maiden bed-warmer. Then there was Ponce de León, the sixteenth-century explorer whose extraordinary quest for the fountain of youth led to the discovery of Florida. And there have always been rich pickings for the devisers of aphrodisiac potions and lotions – anything that enables people (principally men) to enjoy the pleasures of firm flesh for longer.

With the growing knowledge about hormones, the testicles and their hormone testosterone came to be regarded as the sure return route to youth, and for a while, with Brown-Séquard's *liquide testiculaire* storming the world, perhaps it was felt that time *could* be reversed. Certainly, there are many before and after pictures from the early 1900s, of jowly and solid citizens transforming before your very eyes into lithe dilettantes – all down to the restoring power of organotherapy. Autosuggestion and a bit of Vaseline on the lens is more like it.

A rejuvenation boom took place in the 1920s, led principally by the eminent Viennese physiologist, Professor Eugen Steinach (1861–1944). He began a series of experiments on the physiology of the sex organs. He showed that the sexual behaviour of an individual animal is dependent on the sex of the reproductive organs they have implanted, not on their original sex. Thus, ovaries placed in male rats produce feminine behaviours, despite the fact that the rats were male from birth. These experiments were immaculate in their design and conception but were popularized and distorted by the media. Steinach discovered the glandular cells – Leydig cells – that produce testosterone in the testicles; these he called the 'puberty gland'. His experiment – introducing testicular implants into elderly rats – had produced a rejuvenating effect, with previously crumbly animals discovering new interest in female rats and living on average 25 per cent longer. The startling results of this work were all Steinach needed to persuade the world that rejuvenation science was now entirely respectable.

There followed a bizarre series of grafting experiments in which men agreed, apparently willingly, to have bits of testicles from other men stitched into their own genitalia, with the object of rejuvenation or, at the very least, restoration of 'powers'. Donors became a problem, as they were far outnumbered by those who wanted treatment, and implants were soon coming from decidedly dubious sources such as, in the States, electrocuted prisoners and those killed in car crashes. Enthusiasm was fuelled by tales such as that of a football player who had had to be castrated following a sports injury. He received a transplant from the organ of a teenage boy and was said to need an ice pack to control the frequency of erections.

In fact, testosterone has little to do with the mechanics of penile enlargement – it's the hormone of desire and libido, not of erections, which are largely controlled by alterations in the blood flow and the *moment juste*.

Steinach, who could see that glandular grafting would never move forwards while it relied on human donors, came up with an inspired solution. The vas deferens is a narrow tube which carries and stores sperm. There is one on each side of a man's body, taking the sperm released from the testicle on that side along to the prostate gland, where the seminal fluid is added. A single tube then carries sperm and fluid out through the urethra during ejacuation. Male sterilization – a vasectomy – involves cutting both vas deferens before they get to the prostate gland, so that the man still ejaculates semen, but it contains no sperm. Steinach's operation involved severing on vas deferens: you could call it a demi-vasectomy. He claimed that doing this increased the testosterone output of the Leydig cells. The rationale was that since sperm were no longer required, the sperm-producing cells shrank, providing more room for the testosterone-producing Leydig cells. Actually this is nonsense, for sperm continue to be produced after a vasectomy – they just can't exit via the normal route and are reabsorbed by the body. The Steinach operation was performed one vas deferens at a time, which always left the option of a second operation (for a further hefty fee) if the results were not satisfactory. Those who'd had the surgery claimed they felt rejuvenated – a stark contrast to the feeling that men have today about vasectomy. The last thing you'd hear a man saying now is that a vasectomy was likely to increase their sex drive. A typical Steinach enthusiast was the poet W. B. Yeats. He had stopped writing poetry after the death of his companion and mentor Lady Gregory. He decided that the way back to creativity was through potency and opted for a Steinach operation, which was carried out in Harley Street in April

1934 when he was sixty-nine. The sexologist Norman Haire was the surgeon. Perhaps not coincidentally, in September of that year Yeats began a relationship with the young actress and poet Margot Ruddock, who was twenty-seven.

With testimonials from W. B. Yeats and with Steinach thundering 'A man is as old as his endocrine glands', it was perhaps hardly surprising that the Steinach operation became so popular. A vasectomy no more rejuvenates, however, than wearing a hat makes you invisible. The common thread between the work of Steinach and the other youth pedlars who followed him was testosterone. Yet it is hard to fathom why testosterone and the reversal of ageing were ever linked.

The Hormone of Ageing – Testosterone?

The evidence that testosterone is *not* associated with long life is all around us. Women live on average ten years longer than men. Indeed, male mortality is higher than female mortality at all ages. Some of this is cultural – men smoke more than women, for instance, and the mania of early adulthood ensures a high incidence of death by foolhardiness in those years. It is also a direct reflection of the effect of testosterone on the cardiovascular system, which pushes up rates of death from heart attacks and stroke in men. Then there is the evidence from eunuchs. Freed of their male hormones, they live almost as long as women.

Castrati were boys with outstanding singing voices, who were offered by their families for castration as a way of preserving those voices. Many came from very poor families and, although the practice was against the law, these children met with mysterious accidents with wild animals, with their testicles having to be subsequently removed because of 'injury'. They sang female roles (it not being proper for women to tread the boards in the seventeenth and eighteenth centuries) but also male roles since the top parts called for the highest voices. Some, like Farinelli, became immensely famous. The last castrati died in 1922.

Some evidence, too, comes from modern studies of castration. Shockingly, in some US states in the early part of the twentieth century, castration was considered an acceptable way of dealing with those people considered 'unfit' – largely institutionalized men with mental retardation, who were forcibly sterilized in order to protect the American gene pool. In 1969, Dr James Hamilton compared the lifespans of castrated men in long-stay institutions in Kansas with those of age-matched controls at the same hospitals and found a 13.6-year difference in lifespan.

Nor is there much encouragement for testosterone as a youth elixir from the animal world. Some animals have chosen the nuclear option in terms of reproductive strategies. It's literally do and die. The technical name for this is semelparous reproduction – and you are already familiar with one example, the Pacific salmon. They start their lives in nursery ponds way upstream, before making their way to the ocean, where they live for up to four years. Then, in a humbling display of driven determination, they return to their spawning grounds, battling upstream, dodging bears, and leaping impossible heights to overcome waterfalls. The females release eggs, the male their sperm and that's it – they die.

There is but one example of a mammal that has chosen this same option. Antechinus is a type of marsupial shrew. A tiny and rather unremarkable Australian carnivore with a nasty nip, it could easily be overlooked in the grand scheme of things were it not for the fact that it is famous for death by too much sex. 'Way to go' is the usual, rather admiring comment. In late July the mating season begins and the male shrews seemingly become infected with an all-consuming mating mania. They use their teeth to fight off love rivals and also to subdue females, becoming tattered and wounded in the process – though they hardly seem to notice.

Once aboard the mate of their choice, a male Antechinus will thrust away for up to twelve hours, only releasing the female to pursue another. A dozen mates in succession and many for the full twelve-hour stretch is not unusual before they die, usually while still on the job. Way to go indeed.

In Antechinus as in the Pacific salmon, castration before sexual maturity extends life. Deprived of their sex hormones and of the urge to roger anything that moves, the male Antechinus will live twice as long – in fact to the same age as the females. It is a myth that they have more testosterone than adult human males – their blood testosterone is similar to that in other animals of their type – but the difference is that the Antechinus has none of the proteins that would normally mop up testosterone in the blood (sex hormone binding globulins), so it is exposed to full-on testosterone. This is not a pretty sight. Effectively they are doomed to die by their sex hormones. For continued hormone stimulation also means that their adrenal glands are at full stretch too, pumping out steroids. Normally the feedback system ensures that something is done to slow down production. This system seems to fail. Worse, under the influence of all that testosterone, the binding proteins which would normally mop up cortisone are also much reduced. You might think PMT or raging teenage hormones are scary. They have nothing on this.

Sustained hormonal onslaught means that these creatures start to fall apart – their bones become brittle, they develop trouble with their salt balance and become bloated, they get diabetes, their immune system falters, the skin thins and they start to lose their fur in clumps. Shrews don't live long enough to develop cancers, but evidence suggests that they probably would if sex hadn't finished them off first. If you think that these ailments have an all-too-familiar ring, sounding for all the world like the complaints of your granddad, you're right. This is programmed ageing, engineered by hormones.

The concept of a testosterone deficiency state with age has become more accepted, despite the fact that, unlike the menopause, there is no catastrophic 'andropause' in which the level of testosterone plummets, rather a gradual wind-down. Many doubt the 'deficiency' model, particularly given that the level at which treatment is recommended drifts ever upwards, and consider it little more than pharmaceutical-company-inspired hype in which many internet youth pedlars, the silk suit merchants of Harley Street but also men themselves, are all complicit. The promise of improved libido and re-energized sexual activity is a siren call that few men can resist, even given its clear perils. Testosterone has an air of danger and notoriety that few other hormones can match.

Testosterone is powerfully anabolic (that is, it builds muscle), particularly if it is accompanied by resistance exercise. Even a low dose can give athletes a big performance boost, and in a surprisingly short time too, as little as three weeks. Testosterone use (and that of other synthetic anabolic steroids) is banned in competitive sport, but hormone use in sport has degenerated into a different kind of sport, scientists v. scientists, in which those who devise tests to detect the latest anabolic steroid are outwitted by yet more scientists who devise new, undetectable molecules.

There is also a high level of abuse amongst teenagers, anxious to boost their looks or improve their sports performance. A survey of US high school students suggests 3.5 per cent use steroids such as testosterone. Many alarming surveys have shown that athletes would be prepared to trade up to five years of their life, or even death within five years, if there was a substance they could take which would guarantee them a gold medal win.

Steroid abuse is hard to counter when the abusers are teenagers who think themselves invincible and athletes determined to win at all costs. The evidence is that in the short term, the medical dangers of androgen abuse are limited. They certainly cause sterility, along with male breasts and shrunken testicles, while they are being taken, but this seems to be reversible. They also drain the immune system's ability to fight disease, causing a 20 per cent drop in numbers of a white blood cell critical to fighting infection, the natural killer cell. The long-term effects of abuse are more concerning. Almost certainly they include liver cancer, with oral use, as well as cardio-vascular and kidney disease. Colon and prostate cancer are also suspected. Although almost four decades of steroid abuse have elapsed and the long-term effects should now have revealed themselves, they are hard to distinguish amongst the noise of general ageing. Also few will admit to steroid abuse and there is a suspicion that some athletes remain blissfully unaware of the true nature of 'supplements' given to them by their coaches and trainers.

The effects on behaviour, the so-called 'roid rage' which can occur in abusing athletes, are variable in the extreme and some people are much more affected than others. A reduction in empathy is very common, and aggressive, uncontrolled behaviour is often reported. Psychosis is less common. Addiction is claimed, although it is hard to know which drug – exercise itself or steroids – is at fault. The paradox is that steroids can adversely affect performance, while building muscle – a truth which is not generally acknowledged. What is certain is that steroid abuse will continue.

Hair Today, Gone Tomorrow

Nothing ages a man more than the loss of his hair. Grey hair can be dyed, but baldness cannot be hidden nearly as well. Here, too, testosterone is involved. The irritating thing about ageing is that while hair thins on top, it also begins to grow in all sorts of other most unwelcome places – ears, nostrils and back, for example. Women are not immune from this effect either, and they, too, get whiskery with age. Hair on men's bodies is stimulated rather than inhibited by testosterone. Hair on their head can be a different matter altogether, particularly on the crown.

Male pattern baldness – also called by those who want to medicalize it, androgenetic alopecia – is male hormone driven, which, given that testosterone promotes hair growth, seems contradictory. Men who lose their hair in that temples-first, crown-next way, have inherited a gene that makes the hair follicles on their head especially susceptible to androgens, in particular the breakdown product of testosterone, dihydrotestosterone (DHT). This gene is a dominant one, meaning that only one copy is required to have an effect, making it highly likely that it will appear in every generation. At family gatherings, adolescents can hardly fail to notice what is in store for them as they look at the balding pates of their uncles and cousins and see their dad and granddad in all their shining domed glory. It is only of some comfort to dad to confirm to his son that he will be next.

Hair production is similar to that of egg production in women, in that all the hair follicles are present before birth, and there are a finite number, usually around the 100,000 mark. Follicles go through periods of activity and rest before becoming dormant. The hair falls out before starting to grow all over again. Male hormones are metabolized extensively in the scalp and dihydrotestosterone interacts with genetically sensitive hair follicles on the crown and temples. The onslaught of DHT causes the follicles on the crown to become progressively more and more tiny. The single hair that such a miniaturized follicle produces is so fine it can hardly be seen.

Bald men do not have low testosterone levels – in fact they have higher levels of DHT and testosterone in their blood and other scalp hair than those with a full head of hair. There is indeed truth in the old wives' tale that bald men are more virile and likely to have hairier chests than the cranially hirsute.

The key is the enzyme 5-alpha reductase, which creates DHT from testosterone. Bald men have far more of this enzyme knocking about their scalps. A side effect of a drug developed for the treatment of prostate cancer, finasteride, which blocks the action of the enzyme 5-alpha reductase, thus reducing levels of DHT in the scalp, is hair growth and it is now more widely used as a hair restorer than a prostate restorer.

One curious discovery of recent years is that women who inherit polycystic ovary syndrome (PCOS), which causes ovarian hormones to run amok resulting in obesity, hirsutism and infrequent heavy periods (often resulting in infertility), seem to have more male relatives who are bald than one would expect. It's been postulated that the same gene has different effects, depending on gender, causing PCOS in women but premature baldness in men. For some time after this research was revealed, I asked prematurely balding men if their mothers or sisters had period problems and difficulties in conceiving. Many began their replies 'Funny you should say that . . .'

The Goat Gland Doctor

The world will probably never again see the like of John Romulus Brinkley, who made a $12 million fortune from gland grafting.

Brinkley claimed to be a doctor but, although he had spent three years at medical school in Chicago, he had in fact never graduated. Instead, he bought a $500 diploma from the Eclectic Medical University of Kansas which licensed him to practise in Arkansas and Kansas. His early career was spent as a snake oil salesman. He and a partner set themselves up as the Greenville Electro Medical Doctors, injecting people with coloured water for $25 a shot. In 1917, he was working as house doctor at the Swift Meat Packing company in Kansas where he was much struck by the rambunctious nature of the male Toggenborg goats waiting in the slaughterhouse yard. Legend has it that, a couple of years later, a farmer named Stittsworth came to see him, complaining of diminished libido. Remembering the goats, Brinkley is said to have joked, 'What you need is some goat glands' and when Stittsworth immediately replied, 'So doc, put 'em in', he did. Stittsworth was thrilled with the result and shortly afterwards fathered a baby, whom he predictably named Billy.

The stage was set. Brinkley knew of the work of Brown-Séquard, knew a money-making opportunity when he saw one and, as he had already demonstrated, was totally unprincipled. Thanks to Stittsworth, his business was soon booming. Brinkley charged an outrageous $750 an operation, the equivalent of more than $10,000 today. He was grossing $37,500 each and every month. Brinkley was a marketing genius – for instance, saying that his operation was most suited to the intelligent, and least suited to the stupid. This appealed to men's vanity and had them queuing up, proving in the process what intelligent, forward-thinking men they were. He also craftily insisted that patients give up alcohol and tobacco, ensuring that the benifits of abstinence could be attributed to goat glands. Brinkley began to claim that goat glands cured everything from acne to insanity.

Gland grafting was not confined to the US. In Europe, Serge Voronoff, a French surgeon of Russian Jewish extraction, switched to transplant surgery in middle age. In 1921 he too was experiencing problems in obtaining human glands for transplant and decided to resort to animal donors. He preferred chimps, but resorted to monkeys when chimp testicles were not available. His tack was rejuvenation, rather than restoring 'powers'. During the 1920s, Voronoff and monkey gland implants flourished to such an extent that the French government was forced to pass a law making monkey hunting in the French colonies illegal. These implants had a celebrity status in their day rather similar to that which more extreme plastic surgery has now.

The Hormone of Ageing:

DHEA?

There's another hormone that falls significantly with age – dehydroepiandrosterone – thankfully more usually known as DHEA. It is an androgen produced by the cortex of the adrenal glands which sit atop your kidneys. DHEA is used by the body as a general building material to produce other steroid hormones like oestrogen and testosterone. Steroid production starts with cholesterol, and then goes through various permutations on the way to the end of the line, which is oestrogen. One of the 'stops' on the way is androstenedione (known as 'andro' and a common sports abuse drug). There are two forms of DHEA in the blood but the majority of it is in a sulphated form. DHEA supplements can be bought at any drugstore in the USA, but are prescription-only in Britain. They are manufactured from plant chemicals found in soy and wild yams. But please note: eating soya products does not mean ingestion of DHEA.

DHEA soars at puberty and peaks at around the age of twenty-four for women and thirty for men and declines to the low levels of childhood thereafter. At eighty, circulating DHEA is only about 5 per cent of its peak values. This process does not take place at a uniform rate: the majority of the fall is in middle age, flattening out at forty-fiveish. What excited interest in DHEA was some work in the 1980s which showed that levels of DHEA seem to be correlated with predicted lifespan. Also, numerous studies have associated low plasma DHEA with disease – diabetes, cancer and inflammatory disease among others and not necessarily in the elderly. A ten-year follow-up study in Sweden published in 1998 revealed that an older man's chance of having a heart attack was inversely related to his level of DHEA.

If falling levels hasten mortality, then could rising levels extend lifespan? Internet touts were convinced they knew the answer. DHEA is marketed on the internet not only as an elixir for longer life but also for losing or (equally) gaining weight, preventing cancer, boosting the immune system and increasing muscle mass. Given half a chance, they'd claim it can raise the dead and get nasty stains out of carpets too. Given that DHEA is the supposed hormone of longevity, a slight bit of grit in the oyster is that current smokers have a 25 per cent higher DHEA than those who have never smoked. Nevertheless, DHEA-deficiency syndrome seems to be a new term for what most would call old age.

There is some evidence that DHEA is helpful in the treatment of those autoimmune diseases in which the body's own immune system turns on itself. Much commoner in women than men, there's an especially nasty one called lupus, whose main symptoms are extreme fatigue and disabling arthritis. Treatment with DHEA, though not effecting a cure, does allow patients to reduce the amount of other steroids they normally have to take to treat the disease. This is important because steroid drugs have many side effects, particularly at higher doses. DHEA is not without side effects itself and in women has unwanted masculinizing effects, like growth of whiskery hairs on the face, greasy skin and acne, and should therefore be treated with caution. In both men and women, DHEA can cause liver dysfunction. There are also question marks about its relation with breast and prostate cancer.

Like many of the products taken for muscle-boosting, the evidence that it actually does what is claimed is extremely limited. Most researchers agree that DHEA neither raises testosterone concentrations in the blood of men, nor increases their muscle strength. Clinical effects in the elderly are very modest.

There is some science underpinning a theoretical role of DHEA in countering neurological diseases like Alzheimer's but the evidence that it actually has a role is thin on the ground. The most interesting feature of DHEA comes from studies showing high-dose administration to the elderly, who reported a much improved sense of well-being during a four-week study. Relief of mild depression would explain a lot about perceptions of DHEA as a miracle life-enhancer. Just because there are undoubtedly low levels of DHEA in certain disease states does not mean that it is causative or that DHEA is a treatment. There is also evidence from the Australian Sue Ismiel International Study into Women's Health and Hormones, which documents how women's hormones change with age, that DHEA starts to fall far more sharply and earlier in life than hitherto thought, and that significantly it doesn't then alter across the menopause years. In other words, the pretty picture being presented of an increasing fall with age isn't correct. Unproven, unregulated and don't go there is my verdict.

GROWTH HORMONE?

Growth hormone is responsible for growth in childhood and thereafter for a host of body functions, including many aspects of metabolism. It reaches peak production when you are a teenager and thereafter declines steadily, so that the total amount of GH secreted by a sixty-year-old man is about half that secreted by a twenty year old. It is influenced by many things, including age, sex, exercise and food, especially that containing protein. Growth hormone exerts its effects via insulin-like growth factor (IGF-1), which is produced by the liver and by tissues sensitive to IGF-1, such as bone and muscle.

Many of the things that we don't like about ageing – a decrease in lean body mass and an increase in body fat, brittler bones, thinner skin – are also features of adults who have growth hormone deficiency following car accidents or brain surgery for pituitary tumours. These people definitely benefit from regular shots of GH, substantially increasing their lean body mass, and, with longer treatment, their bone and muscle strength too.

You can probably guess what's coming next. In 1990, the *New England Journal of Medicine* (*NEJM*), probably the world's most prestigious medical journal, published a study by Dr Daniel Rudman and his associates from the Medical College of Wisconsin. The study involved twelve men, aged sixty-one to eighty-one, who were apparently healthy but who had (as one would expect) IGF-1 levels below that of young men. These men were given growth hormone injections at a dose twice that given to GH-deficient adults, three times a week for six months, and then compared with nine men who had received no treatment. The study reported a reduction in fat tissue and increase in lean body mass as well as an increase in skin thickness of 7 per cent. Despite these seemingly encouraging results, the study came with a health warning. This was a very short study, there were unpleasant side effects and, the *Journal* warned, nothing was known about the long-term implications.

Significantly, the study did not examine whether the men felt any better or whether they had improved their muscle strength or mobility. Subsequent studies showed that although GH does affect body composition, it does not improve function. The really bad news is that it causes insulin insensitivity, leading to diabetes, there are question marks over links to prostate cancer (a fourfold increased risk) and melanoma, and it can speed up the growth of breast tumours if they are already present. Growth hormone falls with age for a reason – probably because it is protective of some other crucial body function like insulin activity – and it's plausible that low levels in older people are a better indicator of good health than high ones.

Nevertheless, the Rudman study was a call to arms for the anti-ageing industry – prompting in fact, the formation of the American Association of Anti Ageing Medicine, a completely unrecognized branch of medicine. Hundreds of websites sprang up offering oral and inhaled formulations of growth hormone. All protein hormones (and GH is one of them) are destroyed by gastric juice, so oral GH has no value whatsoever, but it didn't stop it being marketed on the internet. If you look carefully you will discover that many of these products are not actually GH at all. A word that is used frequently is 'secretagogues', which is a genuine term for a substance that will prompt release of a hormone. The marketing of these products weaves fact with fiction in the most ingenious way. Here's a typical example:

Product X contains the human unique growth hormone releasing formula used in the famous Rudman experiment. For many users this synergistic combination of arginine, pyroglutamate and lysine is the most potent HGH releaser, dramatically raising IGF-1 levels for a solid eight hours after use.

I sent one such product to a professor of endocrinology, who tried and tested it for me, using his full laboratory kit. There was not even the vaguest flicker of response from a product which cost £60 for a month's supply.

Growth hormone is secreted in response to meals, particularly if they have a high protein content – it's a throwback to our hunter gatherer days when protein wasn't that common in the diet. When it does appear, your body needs to use it to the max, hence the need for a prompt. Arginine, which is naturally found in meat, is given intra-venously by endocrinologists as a standard test of GH function. It should be followed by a spike in GH production. You can achieve the same effect less clinically with two tablespoons of Bovril in a quar-ter pint of hot water. The point is that this rise is short-lived and repeated doses produce decreasing levels of response.

The way that medical scams work is by including some small nugget of truth in the 'sell'. So there was indeed a positive study in the *NEJM*, GH *is* produced in response to a test dose of arginine, and so on – but it's not the whole truth. The *NEJM* found that the Rudman paper was getting more hits on its website than all their other 1990 papers put together. If you click on this reference now, you get a stern commentary from the editor, saying that anti-ageing therapy with growth hormone has not been proved effective and denouncing the way in which their paper has been hijacked by companies wanting to promote their products: 'If people are induced to buy a human growth hormone releaser on the basis of research published in the *Journal*, they are being misled.' Rudman, too, has been forced to publicly disassociate himself from the wilder claims of the growth hormone enthusiasts.

But the story of GH and its disciples is not quite over. In January 2003, the American Food and Drug Administration decided to get tough on the GH-pedlars and sent a warning letter to one company, objecting to their claims that their 'Be Youthful' GH product was effective against depression, fatigue and high blood pressure. In April 2003, another company, Nature's Youth, was forced to destroy

$500,000 worth of stock because they could not substantiate their claims. They cited the Rudman paper as their defence. 'My secret is out, Nature's Youth is how I stay "Good to go and ready to launch",' said the leading promoter of the Nature's Youth product, right-wing shock jock and talkshow host, G. Gordon Liddy. Memories are short. Older people know him better as the man who served a five-year jail sentence for his part in the Watergate conspiracy, which ended with the resignation of President Richard Nixon.

The hype about growth hormone has claimed new victims – who are, in one sense, encouraged by the very people who are supposed to protect them. Athletes, and in particular bodybuilders, have been led to believe that GH is anabolic in adults – that is, it will build new muscle. The International Olympic Committee says it is 'the most anabolic substance known', which is odd because the evidence that short- or long-term administration of GH alone, with other steroids or in combination with training, has an effect on muscle protein manufacture, weight or strength in healthy young to middle-aged humans is very slim indeed.

Women, as I have said, consistently produce more GH than men in response to the same level of exercise, yet they are not more muscular than men. More GH is produced by the body in response to aerobic exercise than to resistance exercise, but it is resistance rather than aerobic exercise that bulks up muscle. Acromegalics, who have very high levels of GH all the time, are not muscular. So why is it so widely believed to have this effect?

Possibly because it does affect body water and connective tissue composition, which leads to greater muscle definition or 'cut'. A bit like vitamins, one suspects that many athletes have a view that you can never have too much of a good thing. The truth is that the side effects of chronic use of growth hormone are deeply alarming – sudden heart attack, diabetes and colorectal cancer. Indeed, all those things that afflict people with acromegaly. Worse, because it is so much cheaper, the type of GH used by athletes may not be the genetically engineered safe variety, but instead the type sourced from cadavers, which is illegal in Britain and many other countries in the world because of the risk of transmission of CJD.

MELATONIN?

A potent marketing tool for many of the modern rejuvenators is the salivary assay. The idea is that your saliva is tested for levels of these various 'anti-ageing' hormones so that an individualized prescription based on your personal 'deficiencies' is prepared. Actually, salivary levels don't always correlate with blood levels and in any case, whether one person's levels can be said to be 'better' than another's is a moot point in itself. As I've said many times before in this book, levels of the same hormone vary enormously between individuals, without any apparent effect on function. It's what is normal for you that counts. Needless to say, these personalized prescriptions cost an arm and a leg. Several legs.

There's another contender for the anti-ageing hormone: melatonin. This is the hormone produced by the pineal gland which is the slave of the body clock. Levels also fall with age. The steepest decline occurs from about the age of fifty, and by sixty, the pineal gland is producing half the amount of melatonin that it did at the age of twenty. In the words of the rejuvenators, 'Not so coincidentally, as melatonin levels drop, we begin to exhibit serious signs of ageing.' Oh really?

Sex is of course part of the picture. Melatonin does indeed prepare many animals for seasonal behaviours. It is thanks to its influence that, in many animals, the gonads increase in size during the breeding season, only to decrease afterwards. So the melatonin pushers contend that taking extra melatonin will keep a man's tackle in unshrivelled condition, much like, er, the equipment of Prairie voles in spring. Also, since sexual dreams are a big part of fantasy, improving sleep (which melatonin may well do) will improve the quality of your sexual fantasy. Pardon?

But the greater enthusiasm for melatonin as an anti-ageing treatment is because it is also a powerful anti-oxidant which, in many different studies, has been shown to protect DNA from damage. It is theorized that decreased levels of melatonin, typically found in shift-workers who are exposed to light at night, may increase the initiation and growth of cancer. One of the first reports from the *Nurses' Health Study*, based on questionnaires from more than 78,000 women, showed that those who had worked thirty or more years on night shifts, with at least three night shifts per month, had an almost 40 per cent greater risk of developing breast cancer compared with those who worked the usual nine-to-five shifts. It is thought this might be because lowered melatonin causes an increase in oestrogen. Another effect of melatonin seems to be inhibition of the enzyme telomerase, which is intimately involved in cell replication, making it more likely that any cancer cell will self-destruct rather than replicate.

It has also been suggested recently that one reason for the increases seen in childhood leukaemias might be because children go to bed later, and sleep with the light on, thus lowering their melatonin and increasing cancer rates. Take this with several pinches of salt, please.

At the moment, melatonin is being trialled as an adjunct to cancer therapies. Some small studies show promise but there is not enough evidence to make any sort of definitive statement. It is also being added to chemotherapy in the hope that it will reduce side effects. Although it seems to do this in some cases, it looks as though it does so at the expense of the effectiveness of the chemotherapy.

The gospel has been that melatonin falls with age but some recent work suggests that this view should be challenged. A study from the National Institute of Health, carried out at Harvard Medical School in 1999 by Dr Charles Czeisler compared thirty-four healthy older men and women over sixty with ninety-eight men under thirty, carefully controlling for confounders which would affect melatonin levels, including the simplest things like switching on the bathroom light if you get up in the middle of the night (which would cause melatonin to drop sharply), as well as drugs commonly used by older people which can lower melatonin, such as aspirin and beta blockers. When they then measured blood levels of melatonin, they found no difference between young and old.

The bad news about melatonin is that some studies suggest high doses could constrict blood vessels in the brain, causing stroke. By all means use it for jet lag – it works well for 50 per cent of those who take it. As for chronic use, there is no evidence of benefit and certainly none at all for clock-turning-back abilities – but there is some evidence of harm.

Having spent most of this chapter saying that hormones aren't the key to longer life, let me now tell you how they might be. The conventional view of ageing is that it is due to an accumulation of random damage, with free radicals – the unwelcome and highly reactive by-products of chemical reactions within the body – the prime suspects. Many of the anti-ageing strategies involve taking vitamins and other supplements that mop up free radicals, although this is spectacularly unsuccessful (despite what you may read).

Radical calorie restriction, however, is known to extend life by up to half as long again in mice and worms and, once again, it is thought that this might work in humans because it will cut the number of free radicals produced over a lifetime. Recent work has shown that knocking out a gene called Daf2 extends lifespan even more than calorie restriction. Daf2 is a hormone receptor for IGF-1, the mediator of growth hormone which, as we have seen, has numerous roles throughout the body, including lessening the response of individual cells to stress. Hormones may indeed hold the key to extended life – in fact, one would be astonished if they were not involved – but we are a long way from even extending lifespan, let alone achieving immortality.

CHAPTER TEN

THE REIGN OF HORMONES IN THE FUTURE

Are You In Control – Or Are They?

You may have started this book thinking that you were in thrall to your hormones. In some ways, you are. Melatonin, the slave of the clock, orders the timetabling of your internal day, synchronizing your life with that of the sun and the seasons. Oestrogen and progesterone, with their rhythmical and relentless ebb and flow, order your cycle and so ordain the fluctuations of your emotions, as well, of course, as the thickness of your womb lining and your readiness for pregnancy each month. The quiet and steady release of growth hormone turns babies into toddlers, into children, into teenagers, and into fully functioning, more or less mature adults.

Actually, the answer must be clear. *You* are in control. For what hormones do is to reflect the brain's – your – responses to change, both those you consciously initiate and those you don't. So if you were to be kept in constant light, or if you were to fall ill and not eat or, as a child, you were deprived of sleep, then your hormones would reflect that circumstance, as the brain – you – decided on a response and sent out the appropriate hormones. This might result in a disruption in your daily rhythms, a cessation of your periods or even a slowing of growth. Equally, your hormones are sent out in response to you tucking away a Christmas dinner, or bungee jumping or meeting the lust of your life.

You manipulate your hormones every day. You exercise, you sleep, you eat. Every mouthful of food you eat contains some sort of hormone-altering substance, whether it be phytoestrogens which dock at your oestrogen receptors and initiate acitivity at a cellular level, as oestrogen would do, or candyfloss on the beach providing a rush of sugar which gets insulin levels soaring.

So, hormones are truly your slaves, albeit extraordinarily powerful slaves. In this book, we've encountered hormones as the cause of trade wars, and hormones as the engine of cultural change.

Life-Changing Hormones – The pill and HRT

the pill, that little double-hormoned package, is the most obvious example. In the 1960s it seemed liberating and allowed women to escape from the drudgery of constant pregnancy with a method of contraception that was in their hands. Today, we wonder if we have misplaced that freedom somewhere, as women are now often expected by men to be responsible for contraception, which, if you ask me, is liberating them not us. Equally, because of the rise and rise of sexually transmitted diseases, we are now suggesting to our young people that the pill is not enough – a barrier method of contraception is also essential. the pill's much-vaunted freedom has been bought at a price, for it has allowed people to have sex literally without consequence, ushering in an era of greatly relaxed attitudes to sex. These have paved the way for our current sexual live-and-let-live mores. This is what we wanted, but did we ever realize that it would involve thousands of teenage pregnancies every year?

Perhaps, however, the pill has allowed us to return to primate-like behaviour. Our closest cousins, chimps and bonobos, are extremely promiscuous. the pill allows us to emulate their behaviour, without the consequences, despite the brain's attempts to corral us to 'the one' with shots of bonding oxytocin.

Hormone replacement therapy for menopausal women ushered in another revolution. Women were no longer consigned to the scrap heap at forty, considered old in our mothers' day. With juiciness preserved by HRT, they showed that there was no deterioration in thought processes between a woman of thirty-five and one of fifty-five and both could be fabulous. They went out, they took no prisoners and they took exercise, watched their diets, looked after themselves. It was all part of the HRT experience and, I suspect, part of the reason for much of the beneficial effect first seen with HRT. For women that took it, HRT allowed them to reclaim their middle years and count them as an extension of youth. And, significantly, it pulled *all* women in that age bracket into its youthful embrace, even those who did not take HRT, shifting perceptions so that sixty became the new fifty. Without HRT, it is possible that this decade-warping effect would never have happened, and certainly, if it had happened, that it would have arrived far later.

Some people say that humans have outgrown their hormones, particularly their stress hormones, which were originally tailor-made for a caveman lifestyle of hunting and being hunted. Surely, having a stress hormone response to someone cutting you up on the motorway is over the top? Actually, I don't agree. We have evolved to survive and to ensure that the human race survives and who knows what we face tomorrow? Our hormones are still fit for purpose.

Where we do need to take care is in ensuring that a generation of children are not blighted by the consequences of their mothers' poverty and despair. For despite everything the body does to attenuate the hormonal stress response in pregnancy, too much maternal stress will irrevocably reset the baby's stress thermostat, condemning a child to a greatly increased hormonal stress response, and to all the consequences of ill-health and unhappiness that may follow.

PUBERTY

Hormones have not been kind to today's teenagers. We have seen how the age of puberty has been falling, linked as it is to better nutrition and higher body fat content. Conditions of plenty have caused confusion, as reproductive hormones course through ten year olds, creating women's bodies with the minds of little girls. Worse, puberty is a time when the brain makes adjustments to those centres controlling executive action, making teenagers particularly unsuited to coping with the adult decisions that they now need to make. In my view, we have to accept that girls with women's bodies are the price of affluence, but we also need to find ways to protect young girls (and to an extent, young boys) from doing things that they will find hard to live with in later years, that push their bodies and brains beyond their maturity.

As for hormone determinsm – in particular that levels of testosterone decide the future direction of people's lives – I am suspicious, yet recognize all the same what tesosterone does show us about teenagers – which is that keeping the wrong company can set behaviour, and turn a potential leader into a gang member with no future.

Uniquely Hormoned

We are all uniquely hormoned. What might be the right level for another person to operate at full function might be wrong for us. There are reference values – numbers which provide a guide as to the top and bottom of usual hormone levels – but these are crude. Moreover, blood levels of a hormone may not reflect what is going on with that hormone at a critical tissue level, which makes knowing how much to put back to restore health difficult. In these terms we are still groping for knowledge. This has implications for attempts at mass hormonization – sales of hormones intended for the benefit of the majority, which may be desperately unhelpful, or potentially even very harmful, to the few.

Hormones are now available to treat virtually all the hormone-deficient diseases. Nor are these hormones full of impurities as they were at first, when manufactured from vast pools of donated urine or from tons of sows' ovaries. Most are produced using bioengineering in a pure, synthesized form or even as designer molecules, such as the new range of insulins. Nevertheless hormone administration is still relatively crude, with most people getting just too much or just too little, rather than providing a complete cure.

If J. F. Kennedy, who had Addison's disease, the disease of the adrenal glands, had been born five years earlier, or had not come from a rich family able to afford the newly synthesized cortisone he needed, the course of history would have been altered. Nobody need die from Addison's disease or insulin-dependent diabetes, or the other hormone insufficiency diseases these days but neither is the idea of an instant return to wellness through hormones a reality. Many patients complain of tiredness or other vague problems, reflecting the fact that replacement hormones are a poor substitute for the extraordinary responsiveness provided by the on-board, in-house variety.

Thus it is that aggressive treatment of over-productive thyroids leads to the reverse problem of hypothyroidism, and the use of hormones in assisted reproduction leads to multiple pregnancy. Some of these problems are now being overcome – for instance, the use of individualized and gradual ovulation induction can assure single pregnancies rather than the nightmare of sextuplets.

There are people – usually geneticists – who claim that in the future genetic testing will ensure better use of hormones, with dosing schedules tailored to the individual. Would that it were so simple. The genes causing many endocrine diseases are just a part of the story, since there is multiple interfering, not just from other interacting hormones, but more particularly from lifestyle choices, so that what you might expect to see from your gene testing is completely different from what you actually see in real life. Reports of genetic crystal-ball-gazing in endocrinology are currently not encouraging. What we will see is genetic testing to reveal disease susceptibility, with the result dictating which of several 'designer' hormone replacement drugs you might be given. For instance, if you were likely to develop osteroporosis, you might be given a selective oestrogen receptor modulator, that acted powerfully on bone but not on breast or womb.

The lessons of the past are that hormones are not magic bullets, with a precise action; rather they are scatterguns. For sure, they may be aimed at one hormone system in particular, but all that we now know should tell us that no hormone or set of hormones works in isolation. All are linked in a fantastically complex web and what you do to one will inevitably cause a ripple effect throughout the endocrine system.

If all the hormones that are needed for replacement in deficiency are already available, what are the new hormonal treatments of the future likely to be?

Increasingly we will see medicalization of lifestyle issues, with solutions provided by hormones and ferociously hyped by the big pharmaceutical companies, hungry for these vast new markets. We are already beginning to see female sexual dysfunction marketed as a disease state which can be cured by testosterone. Recently, patches have been marketed for women, which have been fast-tracked through the regulatory process in the US, although very little has appeared in peer reviewed literature to support their use, or indeed to establish the true incidence of the 'disease' they are treating. We have examined the way in which we seem to be repeating the mistakes of female hormone replacement therapy with testosterone replacement therapy for men. There has already been a noticeable upward drift in levels at which 'deficiency' is said to exist.

There is a fair attempt being made to turn endocrinologists from serious academics to purveyors of hormones aimed at solving lifestyle issues. There are two big growth areas. The first is ageing, increasingly being represented as a hormone deficiency state. The current anti-ageing industry is no better, and sometimes rather worse, than the rejuvenators and organotherapists of the 1920s and 1930s. In this sense, endocrinology has moved no further forward since the era of goat gland implants.

Meanwhile, the second growth area and the biggest lifestyle issue of all – obesity – will make someone very, very rich indeed. Obesity will yield to a hormone-based drug, although it may be ten years before we see it. Yet, while the drug companies are relentlessly pursuing a solution to obesity, diabetes, the most common endocrine disorder of all, which has seen no paradigm shifts in treatment for the best part of ninety years, seems to have been overlooked. When Banting and Best made their momentous discovery of insulin in 1921, diabetes was a rare hormonal disease, treated by endocrinologists. Type 2 diabetes was almost unknown. Today diabetes affects between 5 per cent (Europe) and 7.8 per cent (USA) of those continents' entire populations. Just 5 per cent of those diabetes cases are the insulin-dependent sort, so dramatically cured by Banting's hormone. All the remainder are Type 2 diabetes.

Type 2 diabetes, caused by resistance to insulin, has been heavily medicalized, with nearly everyone affected taking a cocktail of up to eight different drugs over a twenty-four-hour period to control the consequences of their disease, particularly the cardiovascular problems. Yet in a prediction model for the Dutch population, it was calculated that if increased exercise were to eliminate obesity, it would prevent 75 per cent of all cases of Type 2 diabetes in women, and 64 per cent of cases in men. So what on earth are we doing?

It takes no rub of the crystal to predict that endocrine disruptors will continue to be an issue. For wildlife, they are a disaster, but I wonder whether people will be prepared to pay extra on their water bills each year to finally eliminate all steroid hormones from sewage effluent? I suspect not. As for the harms to the human population, the evidence that endocrine disruptors are important is very slim indeed and it would seem that our own internal hormones are far more dangerous. However, this will not prevent campaigners from claiming that chemicals, specifically endocrine disruptors, threaten human health and should be removed. Meanwhile all those things which have a far more potent effect on our hormones and our fertility – obesity, our sedentary lifestyle and smoking – are ignored.

Hormones rule your internal world. Long may their reign continue.

REFERENCES

Here is a list of useful references and books if you want to find out more about hormones. I've highlighted [**in bold**] those that are for the average reader. Science papers can be accessed through PubMed (www.pubmedcentral.nih.gov). The heavyweight textbooks that I used (with a hoist) throughout were:

Wass, J. and Shalet, S., *Oxford Textbook of Endocrinology and Diabetes*, Oxford University Press, 2002

Besser, M. and Thorner, M., *Comprehensive Clinical Endocrinology*, Mosby, 2002

Brook, C. and Marshall, N., *Essential Endocrinology*, 2002 This is a thinnish large-size paperback, intended for medical students, but the book I'd recommend if you are serious about understanding hormones.

Alternatively, the following is cheaper and a tad more accessible.

Neal, M., *How the Endocrine System Works*, Blackwell Science, 2001

If you want self-help books about specific diseases such as diabetes or thyroid, I would recommend the books by endocrinologist **Alan Rubin**, *Thyroid for Dummies* and *Diabetes for Dummies* (both published by Wiley). As for the rarer endocrine diseases, Contact a Family has an international website www.cafamily.org.uk and its comprehensive directory of self-help groups includes many representing those with hormone disorders. These specialist groups are best able to direct you to good sources of relevant literature.

The Endocrine Society (of America) has a large patient information section on its website www.endo-society.org/

The Society for Endocrinology (http://www.endo-society.org/) is the British association for those working in the field. Its website is mainly for professional use.

Rose, S., *The Chemistry of Life*, Penguin, 2004
This is an introductory text to biochemistry. It's very good.

ONE
A BLUFFER'S GUIDE TO HORMONES

Borrell, Merriley, 'Setting the standards for a new science: Edward Schaefer and endocrinology' *Med Hist* 22: 282–290, 1978

Long Hall, Diana, 'The critic and the advocate: contrasting British view on the state of endocrinology in the early 1920s', *J Hist Biol* 9: 269–285, 1976

Medvei, V.C., *The History of Clinical Endocrinology*, Parthenon, 1993

Needham J., *Science and Civilisation in China* (Vol. 6 of *History of Medicine*), Cambridge Press, 2000

Rolleston, Sir Humphrey Davy, *Endocrine Organs in Health and Disease: with a Historical Review*, OUP, 1936

TWO
HORMONE EXPLOSIONS 1: Attraction, Sex and Babies

Amateau S.K., and McCarthy, M., 'Induction of PGE2 by estradiol mediates developmental masculinization of sex behavior', *Nat Neurosci* (6): 643–50, Epub, 2004

Baker, R., *Sperm Wars*, Fourth Estate, 1996

Baron Cohen, S., *The Essential Difference*, Penguin, 2003
Women will want to talk about this book, whilst men will sit silent and brood. It explains Baron Cohen's theory about Asperger's syndrome being an extreme example of the male brain type. Beautifully written, persuasive and evidence based.

Bartels, A., and Zeki, S., 'The neural basis of romantic love', *Neuroreport* 11 (17): 3829–34, 2000

Bartels, A., and Zeki, S., 'The neural correlates of maternal and romantic love', *NeuroImage* 21: 1155–66, 2004

Blackledge, C., *The Story of V*, Weidenfeld & Nicolson, 2003
I love this book, which is a fascinating exploration of the science and culture of female pleasure.

Cooper, P., and Murray, L., *Postnatal depression*, BMJ 316: 1884–6, 1998

Davison, S., 'Changes in androgen levels across the adult female life cycle', Presentation to 86th Annual Endocrine Society Meeting, 2004

Davison, S., 'Androgens in women', *J Steroid Biochem Mol Biol* 85 (2–5): 363–6, 2003

Delbarco-Trillo, J., and Ferkin, M., 'Male mammals respond to a risk of sperm competition conveyed by odours of conspecific males', *Nature* 431(7007): 446–9, 2004

Dickinson, H., 'Sex ratio in relation to father's occupation', *Occup Environ Med* 54 (12): 868–72, 1997

'Breast feeding alters LH secretion patterns', [no authors listed], *Family Planning Today* 3: (1) 2, 1992

Fernandez, N., *et al*, 'A critical review of the role of the major histocompatibility complex in fertilization, preimplantation development and feto-maternal interactions', *Human Reproduction Update*, Vol. 5, No. 3: 234–48, 1999

Fisher, H., *et al*, 'Defining the brain systems of lust, romantic attraction and attachment', *Arch Sex Behav* 31 (5): 413–419, 2002

Gallup, G., 'Does semen have antidepressant properties?', *Arch Sex Behav* (3):289–93, 2002

Gangestad, S., *et al*, 'Changes in women's sexual interests and their partner's mate-retention tactics across the menstrual cycle: evidence for shifting conflicts of interest', *Proc R Soc B* 269: 975–82, 2002

Grant, V., 'Achieving women and declining sex ratios', *Hum Biol* 75 (6): 917–27, 2003

Grant, V., 'Maternal dominance hypothesis: questioning Trivers and Willard', *Evol Psychol* 1: 96–107, 2003

Grazyna, J., *et al*, 'Large breasts and narrow waists indicate high reproductive potential in women' *Proc R Soc Lond B* 271: 1213–17, 2004

Gurdon, J., and Hopwood, N., 'The introduction of Xenopus laevis into developmental biology: of empire, pregnancy testing and ribosomal genes' *Int J Dev Biol* 44: 43–50, 2000

Harder, J., 'Male pheromone stimulates ovarian follicular development and body growth in juvenile female opossums', *Reprod Bio Endocrinol* 11 (1): 21, 2003

Hughes, I., 'Female development – all by default?', *NEJM* 351: 8 748–50, 2004

Hytten, F., *The Clinical Physiology of the Puerperium*, Farrand Press, 1995

James, W. H., 'Hormonal control of sex ratio', *J Theor Biol* 118 (4): 427–41, 1986

James, W. H., 'Further evidence that mammalian sex ratios at birth are partially controlled by parental hormone levels around the time of conception', *Hum Reprod* 19 (6): 1250–6, 2004

Johns, S., 'Subjective life expectancy predicts offspring sex in a contemporary British population', *Biology Letters Proc R Soc Lond B*, online supplement, 2004

Kalamis, C., *Women without Sex*, Self Help Direct, 1997

Lim, M., *et al*, 'Enhanced partner preference in a promiscuous species by manipulating the expression of a single gene', *Nature* 429: 754–57, 2004

Lim, M., *et al*, 'The role of vasopressin the genetic and neural regulation of monogamy', *J Neuroendocrinol* (16): 325–32, 2004

Lloyd, M., 'Birth sex ratios and prostatic cancer in butchers', *Lancet* 561, 1987

Lythgoe, M., 'Is this the one' BBC3 series *Science of love: the chemical bond?*, 2004

Maguire, G., 'Prolactin elevation with antipsychotic medications', *J Clin Psych* 63 (suppl 4), 2002

Manning, J., *Digit Ratio: A pointer to fertility, behaviour and health*, Rutgers University Press, 2002

Milham, S., 'Unusual sex ratio of births to carbon setter fathers', *Am J Ind Med* 23 (5): 829–31, 1993

Neave, N., 'Second to fourth digit ratio, testosterone and perceived male dominance', *Proc R Soc Lond B* 270: 2167–72, 2003

Ober, C., 'HLA and mate choice in humans', *Am J Hum Genet* 61 (3): 494–6, 1997

Russell, J., 'Brain preparations for maternity: adaptive changes in behavioural and neuroendocrine systems during pregnancy and lactation – an overview', *Prog Brain Res* 133: 1–38, 2001

Storey, A., *et al*, 'Hormonal correlates of paternal responsiveness in new and expectant fathers', *Evol Hum Behav* 21(2): 79–95, 2000

'Why do some men experience pregnancy symptoms when their wives are pregnant?' *Scientific American*, August, 2004

Tannahill, R., *Sex in History*, Abacus, 1989

Trivers, R. L., and Willard D. E. 'Natural selection of parental ability to vary the sex ratio of offspring', *Science* 179: 90–92, 1973

Ungerfeld, R., 'Overview of the response of aneostrous ewes to the ram effect', *Reprod Fertil Dev* 16 (4): 479–90, 2004

Wahl, R., 'Could oxytocin administration during labor contribute to autism and related behavioural disorders?', Med Hypotheses 63 (3): 456–60, 2004

Wedekind, C., *et al*, 'MHC-dependent mate preference in humans', *Proc R Sco Lond B* 260: 245–9, 1995

Winslow, J., 'The social deficits of the oxytocin knockout mouse' *Neuropeptides* 36 (2-3): 221–9, 2002

Ziegler, A., *et al*, 'Possible roles for products of polymorphic MHC and linked olfactory receptor genes during selection processes in reproduction' *Am J Reprod Immunol* 48 (1): 34–42, 2002

THREE
HORMONE EXPLOSIONS: The Teenage Years

Apter, D., 'The role of leptin in female adolescence' *Ann NY Acad Sci* 997: 64–76, 2003

Bernhardt, P., and Dabbs, J., 'Testosterone changes during vicarious experiences of winning and losing among fans at sporting events', *Physiol Behav* 65 (1): 59–62, 1998

Dabbs, J., 'Testosterone and occupational choice: actors, ministers and other men', *J Pers Soc Psychol* 59 (6) 1261–5, 1990

Dabbs, J., 'Salivary testosterone and cortisol among late adolescent male offenders', *J Abnorm Child Psychol* 19 (4): 469–78, 1991

Dahl, R., 'Beyond Raging Hormones: the tinderbox in the teenage brain', *Cerebrum The Dana Forum on Brain Science* 5: 3, 2003

Garnett, S. P., 'Relation between hormones and body composition, including bone, in prepubertal children', *Am J Clin Nutr* 80 (4): 966–72, 2004

Giedd, J. N., 'Structural magnetic resonance imaging of the adolescent brain', *Ann NY Acad Sci* 1021: 105–9, 2004

Gogaty, N., and Giedd, J., *et al* , 'Dynamic mapping of human cortical development during childhood through early adulthood', *PNAS* 101 (21): 8174–9, 2004

Hallre, J., *et al*, 'Chronic glucocorticoid defiency-induced abnormal aggression, autonomic hyperarousal and social deficit in rats', *J Neuroendocrinol* 16 (6): 550–7

Hull, K., Harvey, S., 'Growth hormone therapy and Quality of Life: possibilities, pitfalls and mechanisms', *Journal of Endocrinology* 179: 311–33, 2003

Kruk, M., *et al*, 'Fast positive feedback between the adrenocortical stress response and a brain mechanism involved in aggressive behaviour', *Behav Neurosci* 118 (5): 1062–70,2004

Marmot, Sir Michael, *The Status Syndrome*, Bloomsbury, 2004

Mazur, A., and Booth, A., 'Testosterone and dominance in men', *Behav Brain Sci* 21(3): 353–63, 1998

McGivern, R., *et al*, 'Cognitive efficiency on a match to sample task decreases at the onset of puberty in children', *Brain Cogn* 50(1): 73–89, 2002

Parent, A., *et al*, 'The timing of normal puberty and the age limits of sexual precocity: variations around the world, secular trends and changes after migration', *Endocrine Reviews* 24 (5): 668–93, 2003

Park, S., 'Age related changes in the regulation of luteinising hormone secretion by estrogen in women', *Exp Biol Med* 227: 455–64, 2002

Pinker, S., *How the Mind Works*, Allen Lane, 1998
Simply a fantastic, engrossing, wonderful book. Read it.

Rowe, R., *et al*, 'Testosterone, antisocial behavior, and social dominance in boys: pubertal development and biosocial interaction', *Biol Psychiatry*Mar 1: 55 (5): 546–52, 2004

Saluja, G., *et al*, 'Prevalence of and risk factors for depressive symptoms among young adolescents', *Arch Pediatr Adolesc Me* 158 (8): 760–5, 2004

Sapolsky, R. M., and Freeman, W. H., *Why Zebras Don't get Ulcers: A guide to stress, stress related disease and coping*, (W. H. Freeman), 1998

Sapolsky, R. M., *The Trouble with Testosterone*, Simon & Schuster, 1998

Seminara, S. B., *et al*, 'The GPR54 Gene as a regulator of puberty', *NEJM* 349: 1614–27, 2003

Varrotti, A., *et al*, 'Serum leptin levels in girls with precocious puberty', *Diabetes Nutr Metab* 16 (2): 125–9, 2003

Zadik, Z., *et al*, 'Vitamin A and iron supplementation is as efficient as hormonal therapy in constitutionally delayed children', *Clin Endocrinol* 60(6): 682–7, 2004

FOUR
HORMONES AND THE ENVIRONMENT

Colborn, T., *et al*, *Our Stolen Future: Are We Threatening Our Own Fertility, Intelligence, and Survival? – A Scientific Detective Story*, E P Dutton, 1996
Also, very comprehensive website at *www.ourstolenfuture.org*

Cadbury, D., *The Feminisation of Nature*, Hamish Hamilton, 1997

Committee on Toxicity of Chemicals in Food, Consumer Products and the Environment COT statement on adverse trends in development of the male reproductive system – potential chemical causes, 2004
www.advisorybodies.doh.gov.uk/cot/

Cornell University Program on Breast Cancer and Environmental Risk Factors in New York State (BCERF). Wide range of information sheets.
www. envirocancer.cornell.edu

CREDO, Cluster on research into endocrine disruption in Europe, 'Endocrine disruption: the problem', 2004
www.credocluster.info

Defra, Endocrine Disruption in the Marine Environment (EDMAR) Report, 2002
www.defra.gov.uk/environment/chemicals/hormone/report.htm

Durdodie, B., 'Gender bending chemicals: facts and fiction', 2004, Spiked Science
www.spiked-online.com

Environment Agency, 'No going back for sex-change fish', 2004
www.environment-agency/gov.uk/news/821453

European Union, Health and Consumer Protection Directorate General, Food and Feed Safety – hormones in meat, 2004
http://europa.eu.int/comm/dgs/health_consumer/index_en.htm

Fisher, J., 'Environmental anti-androgens and male reproductive health: focus on phthalates and testicular dysgenesis syndrome', *Reproduction* 127: 305–15, 2004

Joffe, M., 'Decreased fertility in Britain compared with Finland', *Lancet* 348 (9027): 616, 1996

Joffe, M., 'Are problems with male reproductive health caused by endocrine disruption?', *Occup Environ Med* 58: 281, 2001

Joffe, M., 'Infertility and environmental pollutants', *British Medical Bulletin* 68: 47–70, 2003

Johnson, A., and Sumpter, J., 'Removal of endocrine-disrupting chemicals in activated sludge treatment works', *Environmental Science & Technology*, 35: 24 4697, 2001

Johnson, A., and Williams, R., 'A model to estimate influent and effluent concentrations of estradiol, estrone and ethinylestradiol at sewage treatment works', *Env Sci Technol* 38, 3649–58, 2004

Moggs, Ashby, Tinwell, *et al*, 'The need to decide if all estrogens are intrinsically similar', *Environmental Health Perspectives* 112: 11 1137–41, 2004

Mueller, S., *et al*, 'Phytoestrogens and their human metabolites show distrinct agonistic and antagonistic properties on estrogen receptor alpha and estrogen receptor beta in human cells', *Toxicological Sciences* 80; 14–25, 2004

Norberg, K., 'Partnership Status and the Human Sex Ratio at Birth' *Proc. R Sco. Lond B Biol. Sci*, 271 (1555): 2403–10, 2004

Pedersen, J., *et al*, 'Human pharmaceuticals, hormones and personal care product ingredients in runoff from agricultural fields irrigated with treated wastewater', presented to 228th American Chemical Society meeting, 2004

Royal Society, 'Endocrine disrupting chemicals', 2000 www.royalsoc.ac.uk/policy/index.html

Sharpe, R. M., and Skakkebaek N. E., 'Are oestrogens involved in falling sperm counts and disorders of the male reproductive tract?', *Lancet* 341(8857):1392–5, 1993

Sharpe, R. M., and Franks, S., 'Environment, lifestyle and infertility – an inter-generational issue', *Nat Med. Suppl*: S33–40, 2002

Sharpe, R. M., 'How strong is the evidence of a link between environmental chemicals and adverse effects on human reproductive health?' *BMJ* 328 447–51, 2004

Shaw, I., and McCully, S., 'A review of the poential impact of dietary endocrine disruptors on the consumer', *International Journal of Food Science and Technology* 37: 471–6. 2002

Toledano, M. B., *et al*, 'Temporal trends in orchidoplexy, Great Britain 1992-1998', *Environmental Health Perspectives*: 111 (1): 129–32, 2003

Turner, K., 'Oestrogens, environmental oestrogens and male reproduction', *Issues in Environmental science and technology* 12: Endocrine disrupting chemicals, Royal Society of Chemistry

Wakefield, J., 'Boys won't be boys', *New Scientist* 174: 2349: 41, 2002

FIVE
HORMONE EXPLOSIONS 3: Hormones as Tyrants

Backstrom, T., *et al*, 'The role of hormones and hormonal treatments in premenstrual syndrome', *CNS Drugs* 17 (5): 325–42, 2003

Cutler, W. B., 'Lunar influences on the reproductive cycle in women', *Hum Biol.* 59(6):959–72, 1987

Farrow, A., 'Prolonged use of oral contraception before planned pregnancy is associated with decreased risk of delayed contraception, *Hum Reprod* 17 (101: 2754–61, 2002

Friedman, R., (ed.), *Behaviour and the Menstrual Cycle*, Marcel Dekker, 1982

Gardner, K., *Premenstrual Syndrome*, in 'Women's Health', Oxford General Practice Series 39, OUP, 1997

Guillebaud, J., *Contraception, Your Questions Answered*, Churchill Livingstone, 2004
Encyclopaedic book, in question and answer format and in my opinion, the source of information on which to base decisions about hormonal contraception.

Harris, C., *PCOS, A Woman's Guide to Dealing with Polycystic Ovary Syndrome*, Harris C, Thorson, 2000
A very good practical guide to help women with PCOS

Henzl, M. R., 'Avoiding menstruation: a review of health and lifestyle issues', *J Reprod Med* 49 (3): 162–74, 2004

Law, S. P., 'The regulation of the menstrual cycle and its relationship to the moon' *Acta Obstet Gynecol Scan* 65 (1): 45–8, 1986

Legato, M., *Eve's Rib*, Harmony Books, 2002
This is an interesting book from a leader in the field of gender specific medicine

McClintock, M. K., 'Menstrual synchrony and suppression' *Nature* 229 224–45, 1971

Redig, M., 'Yams of fortune: the (uncontrolled) birth of oral contraceptives' *Journal of Young Investigators* 6 :(7), 2003 www.jyi.org

Rees, M., *The Menstrual Cycle*, in 'Women's Health', Oxford General Practice Series 39, OUP, 1997

Rowland, A., *et al*, 'Influence of medical conditions and lifestyle factors on the menstrual cycle', *Epidemiology* 13: 668–74, 2002

Shank, J., 'Avoiding synchrony as a strategy of female mate choice', *Psychol Life Sci* 8 (2): 147–76, 2004

Snider, S., 'The pill: thirty years of health concerns', FDA online, 1990

Snowden, C., *et al*, *Patterns and Perceptions of Menstruation: a WHO international collaborative study*, WHO, 1983

Stern, K., and McClintock, M., 'Regulation of ovulation by human pheromones' *Nature* 392 171–79, 1998

Strassman, B., 'Menstrual synchrony pheromones: cause for doubt', *Human Reprod* 14: (3) 579–80, 1999

Symonds, C., *et al*, 'Effects of the menstrual cycle on mood, neurocognitive and neuroendocrine function in healthy premenopausal women' *Psychol Med* 34 (1): 93–102, 2004

Trevathan, W. R., 'No evidence for menstrual synchrony in lesbian couples', *Psychoneuroend* 18 (5–6): 425–35, 1993

Veith, J. L., *et al*, 'Exposure to men influences the occurrence of ovulation in women', *Physiol Behav* 31 (3): 313–5, 1983

Vollman, R. F., *The Menstrual Cycle*, W. H. Saunders, 1977

Weller, K., 'Menstrual synchrony: only in roomates who are close friends?' *Physiol Behav* 58 (5): 883–9, 1995

SIX
HORMONE CRASHES

Allan, C., and McLachlan, R., 'Age related changes in testosterone and the role of replacement therapy in older men', *R Clin Endocrinol* 60: 653–70, 2004

Bandolier, 'Tamoxifen: trials tribulations and truths', 1998
www.jr2.ox.ac.uk/bandolier

Bastian, H., 'Promoting drugs through hairdressers: is nothing sacred?', Reviews (Press), *BMJ* 325: 1180, 2002

BCERF (Cornell University Programme on Breast Cancer and Environmental Risk Factors in New York State), 'Understanding breast cancer rates, 2004; 'Estrogen and breast cancer risk: what is the relationship?'; 'Phytoestrogens and the risk of breast cancer', 2004
www.environcancer.edu.cornell

Beral, V., 'Hormones and Breast Cancer', *Cancer Research UK Scientific Yearbook 2002–03*, 2003

'Soya supplements do not protect against menopause changes', *BMJ* 329: 68, 2004

Boothby, L. A., *et al*, 'Bioidentical hormone therapy: a review' *Menopause* 11 (3): 356–67, 2004

British Menopause Society, 'Termination of the estrogen alone arm of the WHI'; 'Further confusion in postmenopausal health: SCSM message 3.12.2003 on HRT in the prevention of osteoporosis' (2003); 'The Million Women Study and Breast Cancer', (2003) www.the-bms.org

Cancer Research UK, Breast Cancer Factsheet, 2004

Collaborative Group on Hormonal Factors in Breast Cancer, 'Alcohol, tobacco and breast cancer – collaborative reanalysis of individual data from 53 epidemiological studies, including 58,515 women with breast cancer and 95,067 women without the disease', *British Journal of Cancer*: 1234–45, 2002

Coney, S., *The Menopause Industry: How the Medical Establishment Exploits Women*, Hunter House Inc, 1994

Consumer Lab, 'Product review: phytoestrogens - soy and red clover isoflavones', 2001 www.consumerlab.com

Dalais, F., *et al*, 'Effects of a diet rich in phytoestrogens on prostate specific antibodies and sex hormones in men diagnosed with prostate cancer', Urology 64 (3): 510–5, 2004

Greer, Germaine, *The Change*, Hamish Hamilton, 1991

Hoberman, J., and Yesalis, C., 'The history of synthetic testosterone', *Scientific American*, February 1995

Jeffrey, A., and Tice, J., *et al*, 'Phytoestrogen supplements for the treatment of hot flashes: the ICE study' *JAMA*: 290: 207–214, 2003

Lydeking-Olsen, E., *et al*, 'Soymilk or progesterone for prevention of bone loss: a two year randomised, placebo controlled trial', *European Journal of Nutrition* (43 (4): 246–57, August 2004

McPherson, K., 'Where are we now with hormone replacement therapy', *BMJ* 328: 357–58, 2004

Million Women Study Collaborators' 'Breast cancer and HRT in the the Million Women Study' *Lancet* (362); 419–427 [mutiple authors], 2003

Minelli, C., and Abrams, K., *et al*, 'Benefits and harms associated with HRT: clinical decision analysis', *BMJ* 328: 371–410, 2004

Morley, J., and Jacobs, H., 'Male Menopause: fact or fiction', *Medical Crossfire* Vol 3, No 1, 2001

Randal, J., 'Menopause is "by no means confined to the woman" doctor said', News, *Journal of the National Cancer Institute* 94 (15) 1117, 2002

Rees, M., 'Managing Postmenopausal health', *Journal of the British Menopause Society* Supplement 2003

Rymer, J., *et al*, 'Making decisions about hormone replacement therapy', *BMJ* 326: 322–26, 2003

Schultheiss, D., 'Some historical reflections on the ageing male', *World J Urol* 20: 40–44, 2002

Schultheiss, D., 'Frank Lydston revisited', *World J Urol* 21: 356–63, 2003

Scientific American, 'Menopause and the brain', 1998

Taffe, J., *et al*, 'Time to the final menstrual period', *Fertil Steril.* 78(2): 397–403, 2002

Wallace, W. H., and Kelsey, T. W., 'Ovarian reserve and reproductive age may be determined from the measurement of ovarian volume by transvaginal sonography', *Hum Reprod* 19 (7): 1612–7, 2004

Writing Group for the Women's Health Initiative Investigators, 'Risks and benefits of estrogen plus progestorone in healthy post-menopausal women', *JAMA* 288: 321–333, 2002

Van der Schouw, Dr Y., *et al*, 'Effect of soy protein containing isoflavones on cognitive function, bone mineral density, and plasma lipids in postmenopausal women', *JAMA* 292: 65–74, 2004

EIGHT
HORMONES MAKE YOU FAT

BASF Pharma, Reductil: product monograph, 1999

Brogio, F., *et al*, 'Endocrine and non-endocrine actions of ghrelin', *Horm Res* 59 (3) 109–17, 2003

Bulent, O., *et al*, 'Alterations in the dynamics of circulating ghrelin, adiponectin and leptin in human obesity', *Proc Natl Acad Sci USA*, 101(28): 10434–9. Epub 2004

Farooqi, S., *et al*. 'Effects of recombinant leptin therapy in a child with congenital leptin deficiency', *NEJM* 341 879–84, 1999

Garner, M., and Wooley, C., 'Confronting the failure of behavioural and dietary treatments for obesity', *Clin Psych Review* 11: 729–80, 1991

Montague, C. T., and Farooqi, S., *et al*, 'Congenital leptin deficiency is associated with severe early onset obesity in humans', *Nature* 387: 903–8, 1997

Neary, N., *et al*, 'Ghrelin increases energy intake in cancer patients with impaired appetite: acute, randomised, placebo controlled trial', *J Clin Endocrinol Metab* 89 (6): 2832–6, 2004

Ruppel Shell, E., *The Hungry Gene*, Atlantic, 2002
This book, billed as the science of fat and the future of thin is a great read and outlines the history of recent obesity research.

Small, C., and Bloom, S., 'Gut hormones and the control of appetite', *Trends Endocrinol Metab* 15 (6): 259–63, 2004

Staffieri, J. R., 'A study of social stereotype of body image in children', *J Pers Soc Psychol*, 7(1):101–4, September 1967

Wynne, K., Stanley, S., and Bloom, S., 'The gut and regulation of body weight', *J Clin Endocrinol Metab* 89 (6): 2576–82, 2004

Zhang, Y., *et al*, 'Positional cloning of the mouse obese gene and its human homologue', *Nature* 372: 425–32,1994

NINE
HORMONES AS CLOCKS

Barianga, M., 'Setting the human clock: technique challenged', *Science* 297 (5581): 505, 2002

Campbell, S., and Murphy, P., 'Extraocular circadian phototransduction in humans', *Science* 279 (5349): 333–4, 1998

Foster, R., and Kreitzman, L., *Rhythms of Life: the biological clocks that control the daily lives of every living thing*, Profile Books, 2004

Glickman, G., *et al*, 'Ocular input for human melatonin regulation: relevance to breast cancer', *Neuro Endocrinol Lett* 23 Suppl 2: 17–22, 2002

Matell, M., and Meck, W., 'Neuropsychological mechanisms of interval timing behaviour', *BioEssays* 22 (1) 94–103, 2000

Melton, L., 'Rhythm and blues', *New Scientist* 166: 2241, 2000

Palmer, J., *The Living Clock*, OUP, 2002

Rao, S., *et al*, 'The evolution of brain activation during temporal processing', *Nature Neuroscience* 4 (3) 317–23, 2001

Reiter, R., 'Mechanistic insights into possible links between electric power, melatonin, biological rhythms and leukaemia', Children with Leukaemia conference, September 2004

Schernhammer, E., *et al*, 'Epidemiology of urinary melatonin in women and its relation to other hormones and night work', *Cancer Epidemiol Biomarkers Prev* 13 (6): 936–43, 2004

Smolensky, M., *The body clock guide to better health: how to use your body's natural clock to fight illness and achieve maximum health*, Henry Holt, 2000

Wright, K., 'The Times of our Lives', *Scientific American*, theme supplement, September 2002

Wright, K., 'Absence of circadian phase resettting in response to bright light behind the knees', *Science* 297 (5581): 571, 2002

TEN
HORMONES FOR ETERNITY

Barrett, S., 'Growth Hormone Scams', 2003
www.quackwatch.org

Bahrke, M., and Yesalis, 'Psychological and behavioural effects of endogenous testosterone levels and anabolic-androgenic steroids amongst males', *Sports Med* 10 (5): 303–37, 1990

Bang, H., *et al*, 'Comparative studies on level of androgens in hair and plasma with premature male-pattern baldness', *J Dermatol Sci*, 34 (1): 6–11, 2004

Christiansen, K., 'Behavioural effects of androgen in men and women', *J Endocrinol* 170: 39–48, 2001

Coles, S., 'Aging: the reality'; 'The demography of human supercentenarians', *Journals of Gerontology* 59: B579–86, 2004

Consumer Lab, Product review: DHEA supplements, 2002
www.consumerlab.com

Drazen, J., 'Inappropriate advertising of dietary supplements', *NEJM* 348:777–8, 2003

'Medical aspects of drug use in the gym', *Drug and Therapeutics Bulletin* 42 (1), 2004

Fussell, S., *Muscle: Confessions of an Unlikely Bodybuilder*, (Poseidon), 1991
Fabulous funny book which describes what it's like to become a Mr Universe, drugs and all.

Gosden, R., *Cheating Time: Science, sex and ageing*, MacMillan, 1996
This is a wonderful book, written with great style by a scientist absolutely engaged with his subject.

Hinson, J., Raven, P., 'DHEA deficiency syndrome: a new term for old age?', *J Endocrinol* 163 1–5, 1999

Hoberman, J., and Yesalis, 'The history of synthetic testosterone', *Scientific American*, February 1995

Kaufman, K ., 'Androgens and alopecia', *Mol Cell Endocrinol* 198 (1–2): 89–95, 2002

Lee, R. A., *The Bizarre Careers of John R Brinkley*, University of Kentucky Press, 2002

A novel based on Brinkley's life would be dismissed as fanciful. Extraordinary.

McAllan, B., *et al*, 'Seasonal changes in the reproductive anatomy of male *Antechinus stuartii*', *J Morph* 231 (3): 261-75, 1999

Mobbs, C., and Hof, P., (Eds), *Functional Endocrinology of Ageing*, Karger, 1998

Oakwood, M., 'Death after sex', *Biologist* 51 (1), 2004

Rennie, M. J., 'Claims for the anabolic effects of growth hormone: a case of the Emperor's new clothes?', *Br J Sports Med* 37: 100–105, 2003

Rudman, D., *et al*, 'Effects of human growth hormone in men over 60 years old', *NEJM* 323: 1–6, 1990

Schwartz, T. B., ' Henry Harrower and the Turbulent Beginnings of Endocrinology', *Annals of Internal Medicine*, 131 (9): 702–706, 1999

Skerret, P. J., 'DHEA: ignore the hype', 1996 www.quackwatch.org

Takala, J., *et al*, 'Increased mortality associated with growth hormone treatment in critically ill adults', *NEJM* 342 (11): 785–92, 1999

Vance, M. L., 'Can growth hormone prevent aging', *NEJM* 348: 779–80, 2003

Ysalis, C., and Bahrke, M., 'Anabolic-androgenic steroids and related substances', *Curr Sports Med Rep* 1 (4): 246–52, 2002

TEN
THE REIGN OF HORMONES IN THE FUTURE

Lamberts, S., *et al*, 'The future endocrine patient: reflections on the future of clinical endocrinology', *Eur J Endocrinol* 149: 169–175, 2003

GLOSSARY

The same hormone can be called several different names, which can be very confusing. If a hormone is also known by a 'job name' – a name describes the work it does – I've given you this too. I've also given you the US names.

5 alpha reductase an enzyme that converts *testosterone* into a more active form, dihydrotestosterone in some tissues, for instance the scalp.

acromegaly a condition of abnormal enlargement of the skull, jaw hands and feet caused by excessive secretion of *growth hormone* in adulthood. Usually the result of a tumour in the *pituitary* gland.

adiponectin a hormone produced by fat which has a role in regulating energy balance.

adrenals *endocrine glands* situated on top of each of the kidneys which are very important in preparing the body for 'fight or flight'. Also called suprarenal glands. Produce steroid hormones. The outer layer or cortex is divided into three layers: the outer produces *aldosterone*, the middle one, *cortisol* and the inner one, *androgens*. The inner medulla of the gland produces *catecholamines*, *adrenaline* and *noradrenaline*, which are produced in response to stimulation by the nervous system.

adrenaline a hormone produced by the *adrenal* gland involved in the stress response. Its production is triggered by exercise, trauma and emotion. Adrenaline is one of a family of chemicals called *catecholamines*, most of which are *neurotransmitters* (see also *nora-drenaline* and *dopamine*).

adrenocorticotrophin (ACTH) produced by the *anterior pituitary*, it stimulates the cortex (outer layer) of the *adrenal gland* to produce corticosteroids, including *cortisol, aldosterone* and *andro-gens*. Levels of ACTH increase in response to stress, emotion, infection or injury.

aldosterone a *steroid hormone* that plays a vital role in the control of blood pressure and in the regulation of the salts, potassium and sodium, in the blood and tissues. Its 'job name' is *mineralocorticoid*.

amino acids the building blocks from which all proteins are made. There are twenty natural amino acids.

androgens a general name for a family of male sex hormones including *testosterone*, but also others like *androstenedione* and *DHEA*. Androgens are produced by men in their *testis* (95 per cent) and *adrenal glands* (5 per cent), but also by women in their *ovaries* and adrenal glands.

androstenedione an *androgen*.

androsterone an *androgen*.

anovular cycles menstrual cycles in which no egg is released.

anterior pituitary the front lobe of the *pituitary* where many important hormones are manufactured, including *growth hormone, FSH* and *LH*.

binding globulins chemicals that bind to certain hormones (particular reproductive hormones and thyroid hormones), 'chaperoning' them in the blood.

catecholamines a family of chemicals derived from DOPA, which include *dopamine, adrenaline* and *noradrenaline.*

cholesterol a fat which is the starting point for all *steroid hormone* synthesis.

chorionic gonadotrophin (hCG) a hormone produced by the placenta in early pregnancy, which stimulates the *ovaries* to produce *oestrogen* and *progesterone* to maintain the pregnancy. It is excreted in the urine and its detection is the basis of pregnancy tests.

corpus luteum the name for a egg follicle after it has released its egg. Latin for 'yellow body', the corpus luteum secretes hormones which help maintain pregnancy in its earliest stages.

corticosteroids hormones produced by the outer layer (cortex) of the *adrenal glands.*

corticotrophin releasing hormone (CRH) stimulates *adrenocortico-trophin* (ACTH), which in turn controls production of stress hormones. Used to be known as corticotrophin releasing factor (CRF).

cortisol the classic stress hormone. Also known as hydrocortisone. There are also variants called cortisone and corticosterone. Its job name is *glucocorticoid.*

cytokines molecules secreted by cells of the immune system, some of which have a hormone like action.

DHEA (dehydroepiandrosterone) a weak *androgen* that can masculinize but does not affect the function of *testis* or *ovary.* Used as a building block and quickly converted to more potent androgens, such as *androstenedione,* and *testosterone.*

dopamine produced by the adrenal medulla and in the brain. A *catecholamine* that functions as a *neurotransmitter* but can also function like a hormone (for instance, inhibiting the release of *prolactin*).

endocrine disruptors chemicals from the environment, both natural and synthetic, that alter hormone function within the body. Examples include peas, beans and cabbages as well as pesticides and synthetic chemicals such as the bisphenols and phthalates.

endocrine glands glands that release their secretions (hormones) directly into the bloodstream. 'Classic' endocrine glands include *pancreas*, *ovary*, *testis* and *thyroid*.

endocrine system all the glands and hormones of the body.

endocrinologist a doctor specializing in the treatment of hormone problems.

environmental oestrogens chemicals, natural or synthetic, that mimic the effect of *oestrogens* in the body.

epinephrine American name for *adrenaline*.

exocrine glands glands that pipe their secretions to where they are required, for example sweat glands.

follicle stimulating hormone (FSH) stimulates growth and maturation of ovarian follicles in women or sperm in men.

follicles fluid-filled cavities within the ovary in which eggs develop.

follicular phase the first half of the menstrual cycle, before ovulation.

'Free' hormone hormone that is not bound to a *binding globulin* in the blood and which is therefore more biologically active.

GABA (gamma aminobutyric acid) a *neurotransmitter*.

gene expression the process by which the information contained in a specific section of the genetic code within a cell is read, processed and converted into a protein.

ghrelin the hormone of hunger, produced by the stomach.

gigantism a condition caused by overproduction of *growth hormone* during childhood.

glucagon when sugar levels are low glucagon is released to ensure the body's efficient running.

glucocorticoid a hormone, made in the outer layer of the *adrenal gland* (cortex), which has a role in regulating carbohydrate metabolism. The principal glucocorticoid is cortisol.

gonadotrophic a hormone acting on the gonads (ie testis and *ovary*).

gonadotrophin releasing hormone (GnRH) stimlulates *follicle stimulating hormone* and *luteinising hormone* secretion (the hormones that control testis or ovary).

growth hormone a *protein hormone* produced by the *anterior pituitary* with a wide range of effects in addition to the control of growth.

growth hormone releasing hormone (GHRH) a *peptide hormone* that stimulates release of *growth hormone* and *thyroid stimulating hormone* from the *anterior pituitary*. Proteins produced by the hypothalamus.

hypothalamus is the master *endocrine gland* where information received by the brain and hormone activity is coordinated. A cluster of cells, less than a sugar lump in size, it is located in the base of the brain behind the eyes. The hypothalamus secretes a number of hormones that in turn control release of hormones from the front portion of the *pituitary* gland, which dangles from the hypothalamus by a stalk. Those that stimulate release, that are discussed in this book are *thyrotrophin releasing hormone (TRH), gonadotrophin releasing hormone (GnRH), growth hormone releasing hormone (GHRH),* and *corticotrophin releasing hormone (CRH)*. All these hormones are peptides. The hormone *somatostatin* inhibits release of *growth hormone* and *TSH*.

insulin the hormone that is produced by the pancreas in varying amounts depending on the level of glucose (sugar) in the blood. Insulin promotes the absorption of glucose into the liver and into muscle cells.

leptin the hormone that signals the degree of fatness of the body to the brain. Produced by fat cells.

luteinising hormone (LH) triggers ovulation.

luteal phase the second half of the menstrual cycle, after ovulation has occurred.

major histocompatibility complex (MHC) the section of your DNA that carries instructions for a key part of your immune system.

melatonin a hormone produced by the pineal gland. It regulates circadian rhythms. Because it is released only at night, and during darkness, it is sometimes called the hormone of sleep, or the hormone of darkness.

neurotransmitters chemicals, released from nerve endings, which carry messages across the gap between one nerve cell (neuron) and another nerve or muscle cell. *Dopamine, noradrenaline* and *serotonin* are examples.

noradrenaline produced by the adrenal medulla, where it acts as a hormone, and by the nerve endings, where it acts as a *neurotransmitter*. It helps maintain a contant blood pressure.

norepinephrine what Americans call noradrenaline.

molecules the simplest structural units of a chemical or compound.

oestradiol (estradiol in US) the most potent of the natural *oestrogens*. Its full name is oestradiol-17 beta. Also known as E2.

oestrogens a family of female hormones, principally produced by the ovary but also in other sites in the body, such as the brain and fat cells. Men also produce much smaller quantities of oestrogens, principally in the testis and *adrenal glands*, but also in the brain and fat. See also *oestradiol*, *oestrone* and *oestriol*.

oestriol (estriol in US) another common natural *oestrogen*. Also known as E3, it is the major oestrogen of pregnancy.

oestrone (estrone in US) the weakest of the natural *oestrogens*. Also known as E1. It is the major oestrogen found post menopausally.

ovaries two almond-shaped glands, one on either side of the womb, where egg cells (ova) develop. The main site for production of female hormones, *oestrogen* and *progesterone*. The ovaries also produce some male hormones, principally *testosterone*.

oxytocin a hormone made in the *hypothalamus* and stored in the posterior *pituitary*. It has three main functions: in both men and women it is the hormone responsible for mate bonding, sometimes called the monogamy or cuddling hormone. In women, it is the hormone that causes the womb to contract and expel the baby during birth. Synthetic oxytocin – syntocinon – is used to speed up labour. After birth, oxytocin stimulates the flow of milk from the breast in breastfeeding.

pancreas a leaf-shaped organ that lies behind the stomach. It pipes its secretions away through a duct – the pancreatic duct – into the duodenum. Two per cent of it is an *endocrine gland* involved in regulation of the body's fuel system.

parathyroids there are four parathyroids, with two behind either side of the thyroid in the neck. Pea-sized, they regulate calcium, which is vital to muscle contraction, nerve transmission and blood clotting.

peptides a small chain of *amino acids*, usually not more than twenty, when a chain of amino acids becomes a *protein*.

phytoestrogens plant chemicals with a weak ability to mimic the effects of *oestrogen* in the body. Include flavonoids, coumestins and lignans. Found mainly in peas, beans, seeds and berries.

pineal gland a tiny structure within the brain that secretes the hormone *melatonin*.

pituitary the master *endocrine gland*. It is a pea sized structure that dangles from the *hypothalamus* in the base of the brain. The pituitary is divided into two lobes, an anterior portion, which is the site of manufacture of six main hormones: *growth hormone, prolactin, ACTH, TSH, LH* and *FSH*. The posterior portion stores two hormones made by the hypothalamus: *oxytocin* and *vasopressin*. All the hormones made by the pituitary are *protein* hormones.

progesterone a hormone produced by the *ovary* in the second half of the menstrual cycle but also by the placenta during pregnancy. Also produced in small quantities by the *adrenal glands* and testis. Prepares the womb lining for pregnancy and contributes to breast changes.

progestogens drugs similar to *progesterone*, found in the pill and HRT and also used as treatments of some gynaecological problems.

prolactin stimulates production of milk after birth in humans but the same hormone has different effects in many other animals and it is likely that prolactin has a wider role in both males and females than currently understood.

prostaglandins fatty acids that act in a similar way to hormones. They act locally and are found in many different body tissues including the womb, brain and kidneys. They are involved in many body processes such as muscle contraction and inflammation.

proteins bigger chains of *amino acids* are called are proteins as opposed to *peptides*. The point at which something is a small protein or a large peptide is a bit elastic.

protein and peptide hormones these vary in size, from *FSH* and *LH* which are big to *TRH* which is only three amino acids in size. Includes *insulin*.

PYY the hormone of satiety (fullness). Produced by the intestine, it signals you are full up.

receptors the final destination of hormones. 'Docking bays' specific to each hormone which sit either on the outside of the cell (for hormones other than steroids) or within the cells. Following 'docking', the cell carries out an activity in response to the message carried by the hormone. Receptors are not fixed and can appear and disappear at will.

suprachiasmatic nucleus (SCN) the body's master clock located in the brain, which receives information about the brightness and duration of light and then sends information to all parts of the brain that control daily rhythms including, via a relay station, the *pineal gland*.

serotonin a *neurotransmitter* that promotes a sense of well-being.

somatostatin a hormone produced by the *hypothalamus* that inhibits both *growth hormone* and *thyroid stimulating hormone*.

steroid hormones a class of hormones derived from the lipid, cholesterol. They are mainly made by the *adrenal* gland (eg *cortisol*, *aldosterone* and *androgens*) and by testis (*testosterone*) and ovary (*progesterone* and *oestrogen*). Small changes in their chemical structure result in dramatic changes in function.

Testes two testicles, one on each side of the body, which secrete male hormones such as *testosterone*.

testosterone the most potent of the *androgens*, produced in the *testis* in males but also in small quantities in the *ovary* and *adrenals* in women. Powerfully anabolic (builds muscle).

thyroid stimulating hormone (TSH) a *protein hormone* of the *anterior pituitary* which regulates the *thyroid* gland.

thyroid an endocrine organ that sits in the neck, just below your voice box and has two lobes, one on either side of your windpipe, joined by a strap of tissue which makes it look like a butterfly in shape. Thyroid hormones regulate the body's energy levels.

thyrotrophin releasing hormone (TRH) a tiny *peptide hormone* produced by the *hypothalamus* which controls the release of *TSH*.

Thyroxine (T4) and triiodothyronine (T3) the hormones of the thyroid gland. T3 is the most potent. Both are made from iodine.

trophin a hormone that has a releasing effect on another hormone system, eg *gonadotrophin* unleashes the production of FSH and LH from the *pituitary* which then act on testis and ovary.

vasopressin an alternative name for ADH (anti-diuretic hormone). It is also known as AVP (arginine vasopressin). A *peptide hormone* stored in the posterior *pituitary*. It is a very important hormone, regulating water balance. It is also a potent vasoconstrictor. It has another role in the brain, particularly in men, in bonding, especially to their children.

INDEX

Main references are indicated in **bold** type.

hirsutism 119
Hogben, Lancelot 41
hormesis 89
Hormone Foundation 179
hormones
  levels 11
  number of 10–11
  trade wars 101–4
  types of 13–18
  modified amino acids 14
  proteins 13, 14
  steroids 13, 15–16
  word coined (1905) xi–xii
hot flushes 145, 147
House of Commons Health
    Committee Report on Obesity
    (2004) 182, 193, 194
HRT (hormone replacement therapy)
    81, 102, 125, **149–62**, 163, 164,
    180, **238–9**, 242
human chorionic gonadotrophin 14,
    140
human menopausal gonadotrophin
    139–40
Humegon 139
Humphrys, John 156
hunger 191–2
hyperactivity 78
hyperarousal 78–9
hyperglycaemia 186
hyperplasia 152
hypogonadism 177–8, 180
hypophyseal portal system 3
hypothalamic-pituitary axis (HPA) 4
hypothalamus x, 3, **4**, **5–6**, 9, 63, 82,
    105, 113, 177
hypothyroidism 150, 241

idiopathic hypogonadotrophic
    hypogonadism (IHH) 47

IGF–1 102, 149, 230, 231, 238
IGF–2 10
immune system 121–2
Imperial Chemical (Pharmaceuticals)
    Ltd 150
infertility ix, 120, 136–7, 139–40
Institute of Psychiatry 77
insulin xiii, 3, 17, 44, 243
    and diabetes 186–90, 231, 241
International Olympic Committee 233
interval timer 205
iodine 8, 16–17
islets of Langerhans **9–10**
isoflavones 89
isoflavonoids 163
IUD (coil) 118, 137
IVF 113, 139, 144, 212

Jacobs, Professor Howard 136
James, Dr William 38
jet lag 215, 236

Kennedy, John F. 19–20, 241
ketone bodies 186
Kimura, Doreen 49

lactation 6, 57–9
Lamming Committee 101
laxatives 199
Leprechaunism 44
leptin 10–11, 13, 82, 84, 190–96
letrozole 171
Leventhal, S.E. 119
Leydig cells 218, 219
libido ix, 33, 147, 176, 178, 180, 226
Licinio, Dr Julio 198
Liddy, G. Gordon 233
lignans 163
Lovelace, Ada, Countess of 85
lupus 121, 229

luteal phase defect (LPD) 139
luteinising hormone (LH) 6, 14, 56,
57, 64, 82, 105, 106, 107, 112,
119, 134, 140, 177

McClintock, Martha 115–16
McCormick, Katherine Dexter 131,
132, 133
McKenna, Paul 206–7
macrosomia 44
major histocompatibility complex
(MHC) 28, 31
male hormones see androgens
male-pattern baldness 119, 224–6
Manning, John 50
Mantzoros, Professor Christo 196
Marcuse, Max 175
marijuana 205
Marker, Russell 130–31
Marmot, Sir Michael: The Status
Syndrome 78
MC4R receptor 195, 198
Meadows, Dr Nigel 194
meat trade 101–4
Medical Research Council (MRC)
unit, Institute of Psychiatry
77
melanophore-stimulating hormone
(MSH) 2
melatonin 4, 67, 111, 209, 210, 213,
215–16, 234–6, 237
melengesterol acetate 101
Melmed, Shlomo 18–19
memory 206–7
menarche 81, 83
menopause ix, 142–9
menstrual cycle 26–9, 106–8
and disease 121–2
the 'hot romance' effect 114–15
menstrual problems 117–20

menstruating in synchrony 115–17
and mood 123–5
the moon and you 110–11
the statistics 109–10
the stress effect 112–14
metabolism ix, 2, 8, 185, 199–200
metamorphosis 8–9
Million Women Study (MWS) 157,
159, 180
mineralocorticoids 7
Moncada, Salvador 23
mood ix, 2, 123–5
MRC Metabolic Disorders Unit,
Cambridge 191
MS (multiple sclerosis) 121
Murphy, Pat 210–11
muscles 11
myelin 75

National Institute of Health 235–6
National Osteoporosis Society (NOS)
161
Nature's Youth 232–3
negative feedback 5
nerves 5
nervous system ix–x, 2, 4
neural tube defects 137
neuro-endocrinology 2
neurosteroids 125–7
neurotransmitters 7–8, 14, 113,
200–201
'neurotrophic' 5
nitric oxide 22–4
nitroglycerine 23
Nixon, Richard 233
noradrenaline (norepinephrine) 4, 7,
8, 10, 14
Norberg, Karen 100
norepinephrine see noradrenaline
norethisterone 131